ready to...

SCORE?™

you can

AF881104

ScoreCards™ for

Vascular Technology

A Q&A Flashcard Study System for Vascular Technology

2nd Edition

DAVIES

By Cindy Owen, RDMS, RVT, FSDMS
D. E. Strandness, Jr., MD, Emeritus Editor

Library of Congress Cataloging-in-Publication Data

Owen, Cindy, author.

ScoreCards for vascular technology : a Q & A flashcard study system for vascular technology / by Cindy Owen, D.E. Strandness, Jr. — 2nd edition.

p. ; cm.

Includes bibliographical references.

ISBN 978-0-941022-86-6 (alk. paper)

I. Strandness, D. E., Jr. (Donald Eugene), 1928-2002, author. II. Title.

[DNLM: 1. Vascular Diseases—ultrasonography—Examination Questions. WG 18.2]

RC691.6.U47

616.1'307543076—dc23

2015008496

Davies Publishing, Inc.
32 South Raymond Avenue
Pasadena, California 91105-1961

Website: DaviesPublishing.com/telephone 626-792-3046

Cover and text design by Satori Design Group, Inc.

Printed in China.

ISBN 978-0-941022-86-6

CONTENTS

HOW TO USE *SCORECARDS*

As part of our 1-2-3 Step Ultrasound Education and Test Preparation program, *ScoreCards for Vascular Technology* systematically prepares you to pass the Vascular Technology exam for the Registered Vascular Technologist (RVT) credential. It also helps you to master the facts, problem-solving skills, and habits of mind that form the foundation of success not only on your registry exams but also in your career as an ultrasound professional. And it's fun.

ScoreCards covers core concepts and principles topic by topic—facts you must master to pass the RVT exam. At the bottom of every question page is a "footer key," indicating the study topic's place within the Davies test-prep study outline—from cerebrovascular to peripheral arterial, pathology to protocols—so you always know where you are and how you are doing. And at the end of the book you'll find a handy list of all the flashcards cross-referenced to the task-oriented ARDMS exam topics.*

In addition, all questions specifically designed to prep you for the ARDMS "Advanced Item Type" (AIT) questions are identified. This is a new class of question that tests practical sonographic skills by simulating hands-on clinical experience. (See "Examinations and Certifications" at www.ARDMS.org.)

*We use the last best ARDMS content outline for test preparation, updated to ensure complete coverage. The latest exam outlines from ARDMS provide a generalized categorical overview together with very specific clinical tasks, but they can miss key intermediate topics you must know to pass your exam—hence our hybrid approach to study outlines. Here you get it both ways: The table of contents reflects the key topics you need to know to pass the exam; at the end of the book, "*ScoreCards* Questions Cross-Referenced to the ARDMS Exam Content Outline" lists the questions under the ARDMS exam outline categories that were current as of press time.

The AIT questions include three types, which are identified where applicable in a ScoreCard's footer key as indicated in quotation marks below:

- **"AIT–SIC" (Semi-Interactive Console) items**: These questions require the examinee to use a semi-interactive console to correct a problem with the image presented. In the *ScoreCards* system, similar questions are addressed similarly, by asking candidates what is wrong with an image or how to correct a problem. We have included some SIC questions here to provide bonus Physics coverage for Vascular.
- **"AIT–Hotspot" items** require examinees to indicate the answer to a question by pointing at or marking directly on an image. In *ScoreCards*, similar questions ask examinees to indicate the label on an image that corresponds to the correct answer. Hotspot questions appear on the RVT specialty exam.
- **"AIT–PACSim" items**: For reading physicians taking the Physician in Vascular Interpretation (PVI) exam, there are the highly interactive case-based Picture Archive and Communication Simulation (PACSim) questions. These simulate a reading station and require examinees to read a patient's clinical history, evaluate existing image(s), and complete a diagnostic ultrasound report by selecting from the options presented.

ScoreCards for Vascular Technology also contains an image gallery of challenging case-based problems and coverage of physiology and fluid dynamics—the vascular-specific physical principles that you must know to pass the Vascular Technology exam. These physical principles are key to understanding the physiologic bases of the indirect vascular tests, Doppler technology and its clinical applications, and other clinically important issues and applications.

Here are some tips for maximizing the value of the *ScoreCards* system:

Take it with you. The pocket-sized *ScoreCards* study system is designed to be portable. Use it on breaks or between patients. You can review a dozen question/answer items in five minutes.

Study, test yourself, review. As you study vascular technology, *ScoreCards* drills you on key facts and figures, it tests your knowledge of those facts in practical situations, and it provides clear explanations and references for further study. Each Q&A card is keyed to a helpful study outline so that you always know where you are, how you are doing, and how important the topic is to your overall success on the exam.

Triangulate on your target. By itself, the *ScoreCards* study system is a powerful, convenient, and fun way of learning and testing yourself. It is especially effective when used with *Vascular Technology: An Illustrated Review* (Step 1: review text) and *Vascular Technology Review* or *Vascular Technology Interactive Mock Exam* (Step 2: mock examination). Just as each ScoreCard tells you which study topic it covers, it also indicates exactly where in the Step 1 text you can find further information about the subject. So do the Davies mock examinations. This integrated, systematic strategy triangulates on your target. The result? Exam and career success!

Earn CME credit. The *ScoreCards* study system is an SDMS-approved CME activity that can help meet the CME requirements necessary to maintain your registry status once you pass your exams. Use the CME application that follows the last question in this book. You may use the CME application anywhere, anytime, at your convenience.

Check our website. The latest news about your exams, continuing medical education, and diagnostic testing—as well as catalogs of additional resources and online help—is just a click away. Visit us at **DaviesPublishing.com**.

Whether you are a budding vascular technologist or a seasoned cross-training sonographer, mastery of these ScoreCards forms a solid foundation for success. For best results, we strongly urge you to combine *ScoreCards* with *Vascular Technology: An Illustrated Review* and either *Vascular Technology Review* (the book form of the mock exam) or *Vascular Technology Interactive Mock Exam*.

Q 1

Identify the vessels labeled A–G in this illustration of the aortic arch.

a. ______________________________

b. ______________________________

c. ______________________________

d. ______________________________

e. ______________________________

f. ______________________________

g. ______________________________

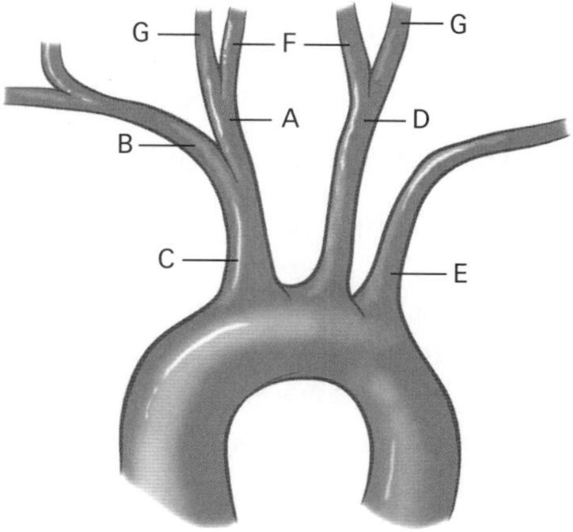

DAVIES
Registry Reviews & Study Aids

A 1

A. Right common carotid artery.

B. Right subclavian artery

C. Innominate (brachiocephalic) artery.

D. Left common carotid artery.

E. Left subclavian artery.

F. External carotid arteries.

G. Internal carotid arteries.

This classic pattern of the aortic arch is seen in approximately 70% of individuals. The first of these branches is the innominate or brachiocephalic trunk, which usually courses 3–4 cm before dividing into the right common carotid and subclavian arteries. The second branch is the left common carotid artery. The common carotid arteries divide into the left and right internal and external carotid arteries. The last branch of the aortic arch is the left subclavian artery.

- Rumwell C, McPharlin M: *Vascular Technology: An Illustrated Review*, 5th edition. Pasadena, Davies Publishing, 2015, p 4.
- Kadir S: Regional anatomy of the thoracic aorta. In *Atlas of Normal and Variant Angiographic Anatomy*. Philadelphia, Saunders, 1991, pp 19–54.

Q 2

The most common anatomic variant of the aortic arch is:

a. an origin of the left vertebral from the aortic arch
b. an origin of the right subclavian from the aortic arch
c. a common origin of the innominate and left common carotid arteries
d. an origin of the right common carotid from the aortic arch

A 2

C. A common origin of the innominate and left common carotid arteries.

A common origin of the innominate and left common carotid arteries is by far the most frequent variant anatomy of the aortic arch, occurring in approximately 22% of individuals.

▸ Kadir S: Regional anatomy of the thoracic aorta. In *Atlas of Normal and Variant Angiographic Anatomy*. Philadelphia, Saunders, 1991, pp 19–54.

Q 3

After it crosses the lateral margin of the first rib, the subclavian artery becomes known as the:

a. brachiocephalic artery

b. axillary artery

c. brachial artery

d. vertebral artery

A 3

B. Axillary artery.

The subclavian artery continues as the axillary artery after it passes the lateral margin of the first rib. The axillary artery in turn becomes the brachial artery.

▶ Rumwell C, McPharlin M: *Vascular Technology: An Illustrated Review*, 5th edition. Pasadena, Davies Publishing, 2015, p 4.

Q 4

The common hepatic, splenic, and left gastric arteries are branches arising from which abdominal artery?

a. superior mesenteric artery

b. proper hepatic artery

c. inferior mesenteric artery

d. celiac trunk

A 4

D. Celiac trunk.

The *celiac trunk* (also called the *celiac artery*) is the first major branch of the abdominal aorta. It divides into the common hepatic, splenic, and left gastric arteries.

Q 5

What is the most common anatomic variant of the renal arteries?

a. retroaortic renal artery

b. multiple renal arteries

c. anterocaval course of the right renal artery

d. congenital absence of one main renal artery

A 5

B. Multiple renal arteries.

The presence of multiple renal arteries is the most common anatomic variant of the renal arteries, occurring in up to 30% of individuals. Multiple renal arteries occur with equal frequency on left and right and may occur unilaterally or bilaterally. They most commonly originate from the abdominal aorta or common iliac arteries but may arise from the superior mesenteric, inferior mesenteric, median sacral, intercostal, lumbar, adrenal, right hepatic, or right colic artery. These anomalous origins of the renal arteries are commonly seen in individuals with ectopic or horseshoe kidneys.

Q 6

What is the name of the tiny intrarenal branches that arise at right angles from the interlobar arteries and course above the renal pyramids?

a. interlobular arteries

b. capsular arteries

c. arcuate arteries

d. segmental arteries

A 6

C. Arcuate arteries.

The main renal artery divides at the hilum of the kidney into segmental renal arteries. These in turn give rise to the interlobar arteries, which course alongside the renal pyramids. The arcuate arteries arise at right angles from the interlobar arteries and course on top of the renal pyramids. Within the renal cortex, the arcuate arteries give rise to the radially oriented interlobular arteries.

Q 7

At the inguinal ligament, the external iliac artery becomes what peripheral artery?

a. common femoral artery

b. profunda femoral artery

c. internal iliac artery

d. superficial femoral artery

A 7

A. Common femoral artery.

Q 8

The dorsalis pedis artery is a continuation of which of the following arteries?

a. posterior tibial artery
b. anterior tibial artery
c. peroneal artery
d. popliteal artery

A 8

B. Anterior tibial artery.

Q 9

What artery supplies the small intestine, right colon, and transverse colon?

a. superior mesenteric artery
b. inferior mesenteric artery
c. gastroduodenal artery
d. left gastric artery

A 9

A. Superior mesenteric artery.

The superior mesenteric artery (SMA) is the second major branch of the abdominal aorta. It arises approximately 1 cm below the origin of the celiac trunk. Major branches of the SMA include the inferior pancreaticoduodenal artery, jejunal and ileal branches, ileocolic artery, right colic artery, and the middle colic artery. The inferior mesenteric artery (IMA) feeds the left third of the transverse colon, the sigmoid colon, and part of the rectum. It is usually much smaller than the SMA. It arises on the left ventral aspect of the abdominal aorta a few centimeters proximal to the aortic bifurcation. Its major branches include the left colic artery, sigmoid branches, and superior rectal artery.

Q 10

The largest branch of the celiac trunk is the:

a. hepatic artery
b. left gastric artery
c. gastroduodenal artery
d. splenic artery

A 10

D. Splenic artery.

Q 11

What is another name for the hypogastric artery?

a. hepatic artery

b. internal iliac artery

c. gastroduodenal artery

d. external iliac artery

A 11

B. Internal iliac artery.

Q 12

Which of the following vessels courses along the medial aspect of the psoas muscle?

a. internal iliac artery
b. inferior mesenteric artery
c. femoral artery
d. external iliac artery

A 12

D. External iliac artery.

Q 13

Which of the following is usually the first branch of the external carotid artery?

a. facial artery
b. superior thyroid artery
c. superficial temporal artery
d. internal maxillary artery

A 13

B. Superior thyroid artery.

Q 14

At what level does the vertebral artery enter the transverse foramina of the cervical spine?

a. C1

b. C2

c. C6

d. C7

A 14

C. C6.

▸ Kadir S: Regional anatomy of the thoracic aorta. In *Atlas of Normal and Variant Angiographic Anatomy*. Philadelphia, Saunders, 1991, pp 19–54.

Q 15

Name the vessels that are labeled in this illustration of the circle of Willis.

a. ______________________________

b. ______________________________

c. ______________________________

d. ______________________________

e. ______________________________

f. ______________________________

g. ______________________________

h. ______________________________

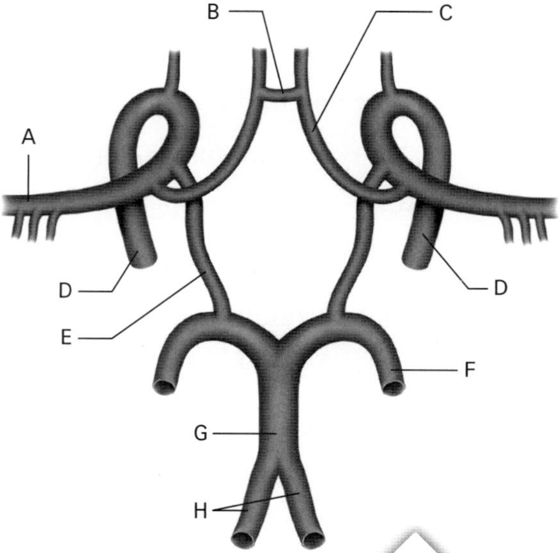

DAVIES
Registry Reviews & Study Aids

A 15

A. Middle cerebral artery.

B. Anterior communicating artery.

C. Anterior cerebral artery.

D. Internal carotid artery.

E. Posterior communicating artery.

F. Posterior cerebral artery.

G. Basilar artery.

H. Vertebral arteries.

▶ Rumwell C, McPharlin M: *Vascular Technology: An Illustrated Review*, 5th edition. Pasadena, Davies Publishing, 2015, p 201.

Q 16

What are the three major branches of the ophthalmic artery?

a. frontal, supraorbital, and nasal arteries

b. superficial temporal, angular, and facial arteries

c. orbital, facial, and nasal arteries

d. frontal, nasal, and lacrimal arteries

A 16

A. Frontal, supraorbital, and nasal arteries.

▶ Uflacker R: *Atlas of Vascular Anatomy—An Angiographic Approach*, 2nd edition. Philadelphia, Lippincott Williams & Wilkins, 2006.

Q 17

The basilar artery divides into the:

a. posterior communicating arteries
b. posterior inferior cerebellar arteries
c. vertebral arteries
d. posterior cerebral arteries

A 17

D. Posterior cerebral arteries.

Q 18

Via which of the following vessels does the external carotid artery provide an anastomotic link to the internal carotid artery?

a. superior thyroid artery

b. superficial temporal artery

c. internal maxillary artery

d. posterior communicating artery

A 18

B. Superficial temporal artery.

The external carotid artery (ECA) can supply the internal carotid artery (ICA) when needed through the periorbital circulation. The three main arteries arising from the ophthalmic artery (supraorbital, frontal, and nasal) have anastomotic links with ECA branches. These connections can provide blood flow to the intracranial circulation in the case of ICA occlusion via retrograde flow through the ophthalmic artery. The supraorbital and frontal arteries connect to the ECA through the superficial temporal artery. The nasal artery becomes the angular artery as it descends along the lateral border of the nose and connects to the ECA via the facial artery.

- Rumwell C, McPharlin M: *Vascular Technology: An Illustrated Review*, 5th edition. Pasadena, Davies Publishing, 2015, pp 199–203.
- Ridgway DP: *Introduction to Vascular Scanning: A Guide for the Complete Beginner*, 4th edition. Pasadena, Davies Publishing, 2014, pp 47–51.

Q 19

Which of the following arteries does **NOT** arise from the intracranial internal carotid artery?

a. middle cerebral artery

b. anterior cerebral artery

c. posterior communicating artery

d. ascending pharyngeal artery

A 19

D. Ascending pharyngeal artery.

Q 20

The ophthalmic artery is a branch of the:

a. internal carotid artery

b. anterior communicating artery

c. anterior cerebral artery

d. external carotid artery

A 20

A. Internal carotid artery.

Q 21

In the presence of internal carotid artery occlusion, all of the following are potential collateral pathways to perfuse the ipsilateral cerebral hemisphere **EXCEPT**:

a. contralateral internal carotid artery through reversed flow in the ipsilateral anterior cerebral artery
b. vertebrobasilar system through the posterior communicating artery
c. contralateral subclavian artery to the internal thoracic artery
d. ipsilateral external carotid artery through the orbit to the ophthalmic artery

A 21

C. Contralateral subclavian artery to the internal thoracic artery.

The internal thoracic artery (also known as the internal mammary artery) is **NOT** a collateral pathway to the cerebral hemisphere. All other answers are potential collateral pathways.

Q 22

Which branch of the external carotid artery provides a collateral pathway to the vertebral artery?

a. lingual artery
b. facial artery
c. occipital artery
d. superficial temporal artery

A 22

C. Occipital artery.

- Rumwell C, McPharlin M: *Vascular Technology: An Illustrated Review*, 5th edition. Pasadena, Davies Publishing, 2015, p 203.
- Ridgway DP: *Introduction to Vascular Scanning: A Guide for the Complete Beginner*, 4th edition. Pasadena, Davies Publishing, 2014, pp 47–51.

Q 23

Which vessel is most likely to be enlarged in the presence of vertebral artery occlusion?

a. ipsilateral external carotid artery

b. contralateral vertebral artery

c. ipsilateral subclavian artery

d. contralateral internal thoracic artery

A 23

B. Contralateral vertebral artery.

In the case of vertebral artery occlusion, compensatory enlargement of the contralateral vertebral is quite common.

Q 24

A 48-year-old male presents with retrograde flow in the left vertebral artery. Which artery is most likely to be occluded?

a. right vertebral artery
b. left subclavian artery
c. right subclavian artery
d. innominate artery

A 24

B. Left subclavian artery.

In the case of proximal left subclavian artery occlusion, the left vertebral artery flow will reverse to provide blood flow to the left arm. This condition is termed *subclavian steal.* Although it occurs more commonly on the left side, it can be present on either side of the body.

Q 25

What is the most common anomaly of the circle of Willis?

a. absence of one of the middle cerebral arteries
b. hypoplasia of the proximal segment of one of the anterior cerebral arteries
c. duplication of the posterior communicating arteries
d. absence or hypoplasia of one or both of the communicating arteries

A 25

D. Absence or hypoplasia of one or both of the communicating arteries.

Q 26

Which of the following is **NOT** a branch of the subclavian artery?

a. vertebral artery
b. thyrocervical trunk
c. brachial artery
d. internal thoracic artery

A 26

C. Brachial artery.

Q 27

The cervical internal carotid artery can be differentiated from the external carotid artery by all of the following **EXCEPT**:

a. The external carotid artery gives off multiple branches in the neck.
b. There are normally no branches of the internal carotid artery in the neck.
c. A bulbous area is seen at the origin of the internal carotid artery.
d. The internal carotid artery is usually located anteromedial to the external carotid artery.

A 27

D. This statement–"the internal carotid artery is usually located anteromedial to the external carotid artery"–is **NOT** true.

The internal carotid artery is usually located lateral and posterior to the external carotid artery.

Q 28

Which of these vessels joins the brachial veins to form the axillary vein?

a. innominate vein

b. subclavian vein

c. basilic vein

d. cephalic vein

A 28

C. Basilic vein.

The basilic vein is a superficial vein of the upper extremity that joins with the brachial veins to form the axillary vein. It begins on the ulnar side of the forearm and crosses ventrally at the antecubital region. The basilic vein lies medial to the brachial artery in the upper arm.

▶ Rumwell C, McPharlin M: *Vascular Technology: An Illustrated Review*, 5th edition. Pasadena, Davies Publishing, 2015, pp 272–273.

Q 29

Which vein in the antecubital fossa connects the cephalic and basilic veins?

a. axillary vein
b. cephalic vein
c. median cubital vein
d. basilic vein

A 29

C. Median cubital vein.

Q 30

Which of the following is **NOT** a deep vein of the upper extremity?

a. cephalic vein

b. axillary vein

c. brachial vein

d. radial vein

A 30

A. Cephalic vein.

The deep veins of the upper extremity include the deep palmar venous arch, radial veins, ulnar veins and interosseous veins of the forearm, brachial veins, and axillary vein. The deep veins accompany the same-named arteries and are usually paired. The cephalic, basilic, and median cubital veins are superficial veins. They do not accompany an artery and are not paired.

▶ Rumwell C, McPharlin M: *Vascular Technology: An Illustrated Review*, 5th edition. Pasadena, Davies Publishing, 2015, p 272.

Q 31

Where is the brachiocephalic vein found?

a. only on the right side of the neck

b. only on the left side of the neck

c. There is no such vein.

d. on both the right and left sides of the neck

A 31

D. On both the right and left sides of the neck.

The venous anatomy of the neck differs from the arterial anatomy in that the brachiocephalic vein occurs bilaterally, whereas the brachiocephalic (innominate) artery is found only on the right side. The brachiocephalic vein is formed by the junction of the subclavian and internal jugular veins.

Q 32

What is the longest vein in the body?

a. great saphenous vein

b. posterior tibial vein

c. basilic vein

d. femoral vein

A 32

A. Great saphenous vein.

Q 33

Which of the following is **NOT** true regarding perforating veins?

a. They direct blood from the deep system into the superficial system.
b. They have one valve each.
c. They are more numerous in the calf than in the thigh.
d. They are known as varicose veins when they are tortuous and dilated due to incompetent valves.

A 33

A. This statement–"they direct blood from the deep system into the superficial system"–is **NOT** true.

Perforating veins do **NOT** direct blood from the deep system into the superficial system. They direct blood flow from the superficial system (great and small saphenous veins) into the deep system. All of the other statements are true.

- Rumwell C, McPharlin M: *Vascular Technology: An Illustrated Review*, 5th edition. Pasadena, Davies Publishing, 2015, pp 269–270.

Q 34

The portal vein is formed by the junction of which of the following veins?

a. superior mesenteric and left gastric veins
b. splenic and superior mesenteric veins
c. inferior mesenteric and splenic veins
d. umbilical and splenic veins

A 34

B. Splenic and superior mesenteric veins.

Q 35

The vein that normally courses between the superior mesenteric artery and the abdominal aorta is the:

a. portal vein

b. superior mesenteric vein

c. inferior mesenteric vein

d. left renal vein

A 35

D. Left renal vein.

The normal course of the left renal vein is between the abdominal aorta and the superior mesenteric artery. Rarely, it may course behind the abdominal aorta as a retroaortic left renal vein, or it may form a ring around the aorta as a circumaortic left renal vein.

Q 36

Which statement is **NOT** true regarding the soleal veins?

a. They empty into the posterior tibial or peroneal veins.
b. They connect with the superficial venous system.
c. They are found deep in the calf muscle.
d. They do not contain valves.

A 36

B. This statement—"they connect with the superficial venous system"—is **NOT** true.

The soleal veins do **NOT** connect with the superficial venous system of the leg.

▶ Rumwell C, McPharlin M: *Vascular Technology: An Illustrated Review*, 5th edition. Pasadena, Davies Publishing, 2015, p 269.

Q 37

Which veins are connected to the gastrocnemius veins by the paratibial perforating veins?

a. posterior tibial veins

b. anterior tibial veins

c. peroneal veins

d. popliteal veins

A 37

A. Posterior tibial veins.

In the leg, there are 16 constant perforating veins. Eight of these drain into the posterior tibial veins. These are known as *paratibial perforators* (formerly *Boyd's veins*) and *posterior tibial perforators* (formerly *Cockett's veins*). There are 4 perforating veins that drain into the peroneal veins and 4 that drain into the soleal and genicular veins. In the thigh, there are 2 constant perforating veins. These are known as *femoral canal perforators* (formerly *Dodd's group* or the *perforating veins of Hunter*).

Note: In 2003 the International Union of Phlebology issued guidelines for venous nomenclature. The nomenclature for *Boyd's* and *Cockett's perforators* is now *paratibial perforators* and *posterior tibial perforators*, respectively. The nomenclature for the *Dodd's* or *Hunterian perforators* is now *femoral canal perforators*.

▶ Uflacker R: *Atlas of Vascular Anatomy—An Angiographic Approach*, 2nd edition. Philadelphia, Lippincott Williams & Wilkins, 2006.

Q 38

The splenic vein drains into the:

a. inferior vena cava

b. hepatic vein

c. superior mesenteric vein

d. portal vein

A 38

D. Portal vein.

Q 39

The hepatic veins drain into the:

a. inferior vena cava
b. portal veins
c. hepatic arteries
d. superior mesenteric vein

A 39

A. Inferior vena cava.

Q 40

All of these statements about the inferior vena cava are true **EXCEPT**:

a. The inferior vena cava has no valves below the level of its insertion into the heart.

b. The inferior vena cava is formed by the confluence of the common iliac veins.

c. The inferior vena cava drains into the left atrium of the heart.

d. The inferior vena cava courses to the right of the abdominal aorta.

A 40

C. This statement–"the IVC drains into the left atrium of the heart"–is **NOT** true.

The IVC drains into the RIGHT atrium of the heart.

Q 41

What is the term for the outermost layer of the arterial wall?

a. intima

b. media

c. adventitia

d. fascia

A 41

C. Adventitia.

The three layers of the arterial wall from the outermost to the innermost are the adventitia, media, and intima.

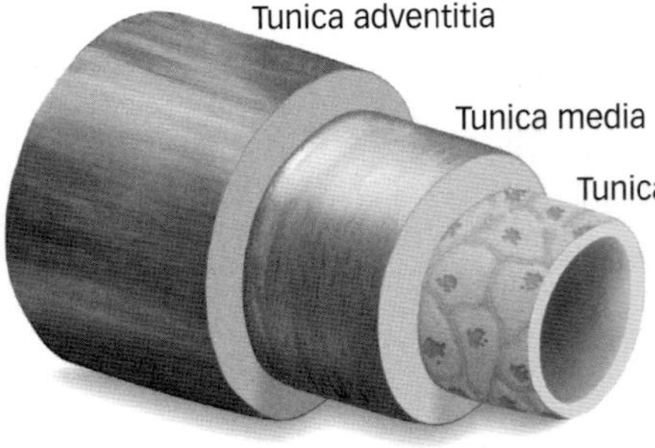

Q 42

What is the primary function of the vasa vasorum?

a. to regulate vasodilatation of the arterioles
b. to provide nourishment to the tunica adventitia
c. to provide the major communication in arteriovenous fistulas
d. to provide autoregulation of blood flow to the brain

A 42

B. To provide nourishment to the tunica adventitia.

- Rumwell C, McPharlin M: *Vascular Technology: An Illustrated Review*, 5th edition. Pasadena, Davies Publishing, 2015, p 204.
- Belanger AC: *Vascular Anatomy and Physiology*. Pasadena, Davies Publishing, 1999, p 25.

Q 43

What is the function of the bicuspid valves of the veins?

a. to maintain unidirectional flow within the venous system
b. to provide nourishment to the tunica intima
c. to prevent communication between arteries and veins
d. to direct the flow of blood away from the heart

A 43

A. To maintain unidirectional flow within the venous system.

The bicuspid valves of the veins are designed to direct the flow of blood back toward the heart by closing during retrograde flow. These valves are sometimes called *semilunar valves* because they appear crescent-shaped.

- Rumwell C, McPharlin M: *Vascular Technology: An Illustrated Review*, 5th edition. Pasadena, Davies Publishing, 2015, pp 275–276.
- Belanger AC: *Vascular Anatomy and Physiology*. Pasadena, Davies Publishing, 1999, p 177–179.

Q 44

The greatest number of valves is found in which of the following veins?

a. femoral vein

b. common femoral vein

c. popliteal vein

d. great saphenous vein

A 44

D. Great saphenous vein (GSV).

The GSV typically has 10–12 valves throughout its length. The numbers of valves in other major veins are listed below:

- small saphenous, 6–12
- soleal sinuses, none
- perforators, 1 valve each; large perforators, up to 3
- infrapopliteal (deep veins), 7–12 valves each
- popliteal and femoral, 1–3 valves each; deep system has an average of 5 between inguinal ligament and posterior fossa
- common femoral, 1 valve
- external iliac has valves only about 25% of the time
- common iliac, none
- internal iliac, none
- inferior vena cava, none
- internal jugular vein, 1 valve

▶ Rumwell C, McPharlin M: *Vascular Technology: An Illustrated Review*, 5th edition. Pasadena, Davies Publishing, 2015, p 276.

Q 45

The bicuspid valves of the venous system are formed by folds of the:

a. adventitia

b. intima

c. media

d. smooth muscle fibers

A 45

B. Intima.

The venous valves are formed by folds of the venous intimal epithelium.

▶ Uflacker R: *Atlas of Vascular Anatomy—An Angiographic Approach*, 2nd edition. Philadelphia, Lippincott Williams & Wilkins, 2006.

Q 46

Which are the smallest vessels in the body?

a. arterioles

b. venules

c. capillaries

d. intimas

A 46

C. Capillaries.

As arteries divide and become smaller and smaller they shed their outermost coat (adventitia) and become two-layered vessels known as arterioles. As they extend further toward the periphery, they shed the tunic media and become submillimeter in diameter. They are then single-walled vessels known as capillaries.

▶ Belanger AC: *Vascular Anatomy and Physiology*. Pasadena, Davies Publishing, 1999, pp 25–29.

Q 47

What is demonstrated by helical flow with flow separation in the posterolateral aspect of the carotid bulb?

a. normal flow dynamics

b. dissection

c. stenosis

d. thrombosis

A 47

A. Normal flow dynamics.

Flow separation at the posterior wall of the carotid bulb occurs because the linear momentum of the flow is disrupted by the large sinus and sharp curve at the carotid bulb. Pressure is higher and velocity lower at the point of flow separation. Flow separation depends on a relatively disease-free bulb.

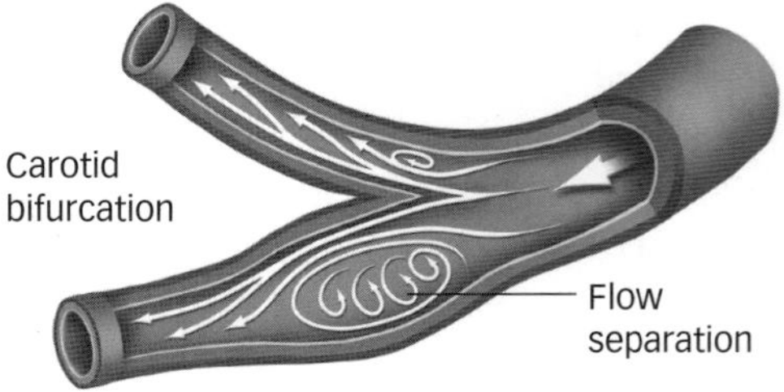

Hemodynamic principle:
↓ Velocity ↑ Pressure

- Rumwell C, McPharlin M: *Vascular Technology: An Illustrated Review*, 5th edition. Pasadena, Davies Publishing, 2015, p 26.
- Ku DN, Lumsden A: Blood flow patterns in cerebrovascular disease. In Bernstein EF (ed): *Noninvasive Diagnostic Techniques in Vascular Disease*, 3rd edition. St. Louis, Mosby, 1985, pp 73–83.

Q 48

What does the Reynolds number describe?

a. the pressure drop across a hemodynamically significant stenosis

b. the flow acceleration through a stenosis

c. the dampened flow proximal to a stenosis

d. the point at which flow becomes turbulent

A 48

D. The point at which flow becomes turbulent.

The equation for the Reynolds number is $RE = V\rho 2r \div \eta$ where RE = Reynolds number, V = velocity, ρ = fluid density, r = vessel radius, and η = fluid viscosity. Turbulence begins to occur when RE exceeds 2000. Since fluid density and viscosity are constant for a given patient, the factors most responsible for creating turbulence are velocity and vessel radius.

▸ Rumwell C, McPharlin M: *Vascular Technology: An Illustrated Review*, 5th edition. Pasadena, Davies Publishing, 2015, p 24.

Q 49

This spectrum was obtained with a small sample volume from the center of the internal carotid artery. Which term can be used to describe the flow depicted by this waveform?

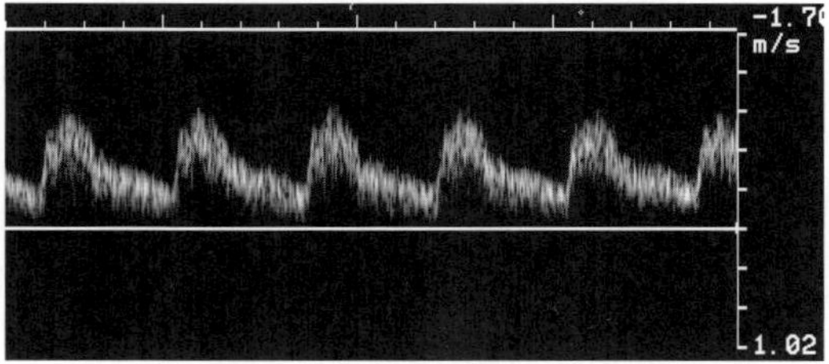

a. laminar

b. poststenotic turbulence

c. stenotic jet

d. tardus parvus

DAVIES
Registry Reviews & Study Aids

A 49

A. Laminar.

Laminar flow is characterized as normal, nonturbulent flow in which the blood tends to course in layers of decreasing speed from the center streamline toward the vessel wall. Laminar flow in small vessels assumes a parabolic flow profile. In larger vessels such as the common carotid artery, laminar flow assumes a more blunted or "plug" flow profile at systole and a parabolic flow profile at diastole.

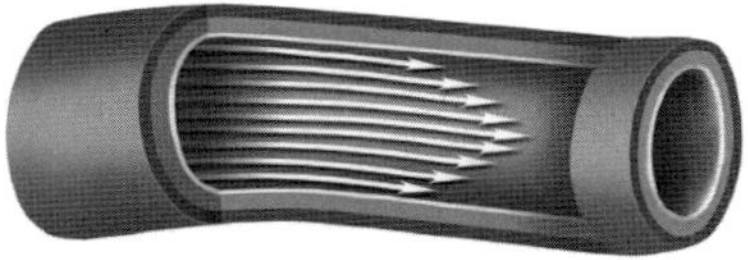

- Rumwell C, McPharlin M: *Vascular Technology: An Illustrated Review*, 5th edition. Pasadena, Davies Publishing, 2015, pp 20–21.
- Belanger AC: *Vascular Anatomy and Physiology*. Pasadena, Davies Publishing, 1999, pp 117–125.

Q 50

Which abdominal vein normally exhibits a pulsatile (bidirectional) waveform?

a. splenic vein
b. superior mesenteric vein
c. portal vein
d. hepatic vein

A 50

D. Hepatic vein.

Normally, hepatic venous flow is hepatofugal (away from the liver) and typically bidirectional (pulsatile) because it flows into the IVC. Renal venous flow, which also moves into the IVC, is similarly pulsatile. In comparison, the hepatopetal (toward the liver) flow of the superior mesenteric, splenic, and portal veins is characteristically phasic and continuous.

▶ Rumwell C, McPharlin M: *Vascular Technology: An Illustrated Review*, 5th edition. Pasadena, Davies Publishing, 2015, pp 319–320.

Q 51

Normal flow in the portal vein is described as:

a. hepatofugal

b. hepatopetal

c. bidirectional

d. triphasic

A 51

B. Hepatopetal.

Blood in the portal vein normally flows toward and into the liver. This flow direction is termed *hepatopetal.* The term *hepatofugal* describes flow coursing away from the liver in the portal vein and is a sign of advanced portal hypertension.

Q 52

The normal waveform of the hepatic veins can be described as:

a. pulsatile

b. continuous

c. unidirectional

d. b and c

A 52

A. Pulsatile.

Doppler spectra showing the normal pulsatile flow of the hepatic vein (A) compared to the phasic, continuous flow of the portal vein (B).

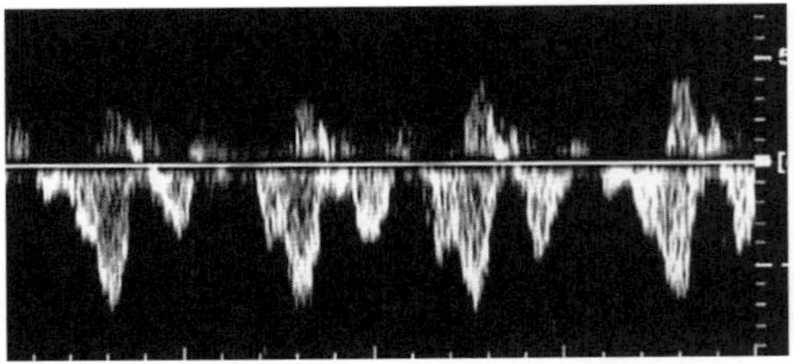

A

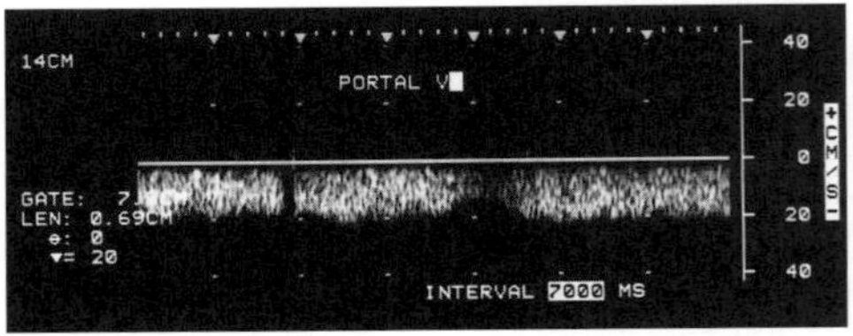

B

▸ Rumwell C, McPharlin M: *Vascular Technology: An Illustrated Review*, 5th edition. Pasadena, Davies Publishing, 2015, pp 319–320.

Q 53

Which of the following veins is **NOT** a paired vein?

a. radial

b. posterior tibial

c. peroneal

d. cephalic

A 53

D. Cephalic.

Q 54

The basilic vein is best described as:

a. a large single vein located near the brachial veins
b. a small vein located deep within the calf muscle
c. a very small vein that joins the subclavian vein
d. a large vein coursing lateral to the cephalic vein

A 54

A. A large single vein located near the brachial veins.

Q 55

The renal arteries arise from the abdominal aorta approximately 1 cm distal to the:

a. inferior mesenteric artery

b. left gastric artery

c. superior mesenteric artery

d. celiac trunk

A 55

C. Superior mesenteric artery.

Q 56

Identify the vessels labeled A–L in this illustration of the abdominal arteries.

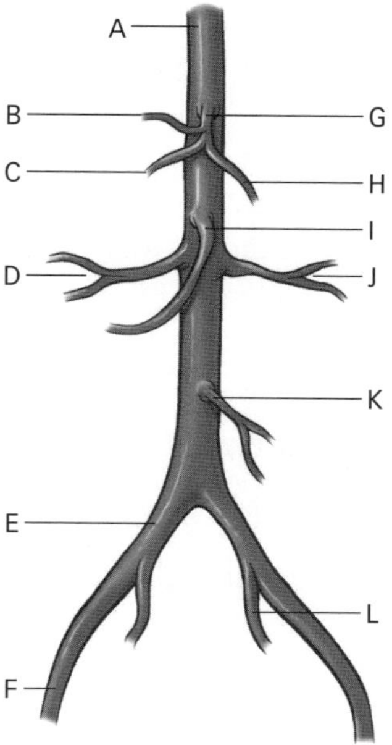

a. ____________________ g. ____________________

b. ____________________ h. ____________________

c. ____________________ i. ____________________

d. ____________________ j. ____________________

e. ____________________ k. ____________________

f. ____________________ l. ____________________

A 56

A. Abdominal aorta.

B. Left gastric artery.

C. Common hepatic artery.

D. Right renal artery.

E. Common iliac artery.

F. External iliac artery.

G. Celiac trunk.

H. Splenic artery.

I. Super mesenteric artery.

J. Left renal artery.

K. Inferior mesenteric artery.

L. Internal iliac artery.

▶ Rumwell C, McPharlin M: *Vascular Technology: An Illustrated Review*, 5th edition. Pasadena, Davies Publishing, 2015, p 9.

Q 57

What is the most prevalent type of stroke?

a. ischemic

b. hemorrhagic

c. septic embolic

d. venous thrombotic

A 57

A. Ischemic.

Approximately 85% of strokes are ischemic in origin, with only 15% of strokes being due to intracerebral hemorrhage. Strokes caused by hemorrhage, however, account for most stroke fatalities.

- American Heart Association: About stroke. Available at http://www.strokeassociation.org/STROKEORG/AboutStroke/TypesofStroke/Types-of-Stroke_UCM_308531_SubHomePage.jsp.

Q 58

Which of the following is **NOT** considered to be a risk factor for the development of stroke?

a. cigarette smoking

b. female gender

c. diabetes mellitus

d. cardiac arrhythmia

A 58

B. Female gender.

Predisposing factors for stroke include male sex, age over 55, cigarette smoking, alcohol abuse, hypertension, diabetes mellitus, hyperlipidemia, coronary artery disease, and cardiac arrhythmia.

▸ Rumwell C, McPharlin M: *Vascular Technology: An Illustrated Review*, 5th edition. Pasadena, Davies Publishing, 2015, p 210.

Q 59

Where would a carotid body tumor be located?

a. within the internal jugular vein
b. medial to the origin of the external carotid artery
c. between the internal and external carotid arteries
d. in the submandibular gland

A 59

C. Between the internal and external carotid arteries.

Q 60

What is the term for a fragment of atherosclerotic debris that courses distal through the vasculature until it lodges in a small vessel?

a. thrombus

b. dissection

c. hematoma

d. embolus

A 60

D. Embolus.

Q 61

Which vessel or vessels provide the primary arterial supply to carotid body tumors?

a. vertebral artery

b. thyrocervical trunk

c. vasa vasorum of the internal carotid artery

d. branches of the external carotid artery

A 61

D. Branches of the external carotid artery.

Q 62

In which of the following vessels will flow reverse secondary to innominate artery occlusion?

a. right vertebral artery

b. right common carotid artery

c. left vertebral artery

d. both a and b

DAVIES
Registry Reviews & Study Aids

A 62

D. Both A and B.

In the case of innominate artery occlusion, flow in the ipsilateral (right) vertebral artery will reverse to provide blood flow to the arm. If the vertebral artery can carry a sufficient volume of blood flow, carotid recovery will occur. With carotid recovery, some of the reversed flow in the vertebral artery will course to the common carotid artery, providing it with antegrade flow. If this is the case, the waveform profile in the common carotid will be dampened with a delay in the systolic rise time. If carotid recovery does not occur, the flow in the common carotid artery will be either bidirectional or completely retrograde, providing additional flow to the right subclavian artery. In this case the common carotid usually receives its blood supply from the ipsilateral external carotid artery.

Q 63

What is the biggest controllable risk factor for stroke?

a. hypercholesterolemia

b. hypertension

c. sedentary life style

d. alcohol abuse

A 63

B. Hypertension.

Effective control of hypertension can decrease the risk of stroke by about 42%. The higher the blood pressure, the greater the risk for stroke.

- American Stroke Association: Stroke risk factors. http://www.strokeassociation.org/STROKEORG/AboutStroke/UnderstandingRisk/Understanding-Stroke-Risk_UCM_308539_SubHomePage.jsp.
- Kelley RE: Stroke prevention and intervention. Postgraduate Medicine 103:43–62, 1998.

Q 64

All of the following statements regarding subclavian steal are true **EXCEPT**:

a. Subclavian steal results from severe stenosis or occlusion of the proximal vertebral artery.

b. Subclavian steal most commonly occurs on the left side.

c. Most patients are asymptomatic.

d. In the presence of subclavian steal, lower blood pressure is seen in the affected arm.

A 64

A. This statement–"subclavian steal results from severe stenosis or occlusion of the proximal vertebral artery"–is **NOT** true.

All the other statements are correct. In subclavian steal, a severe stenosis or occlusion is present in the proximal subclavian artery. This results in retrograde flow in the ipsilateral vertebral artery. The flow is "stolen" from the contralateral vertebral artery by way of the basilar artery. Although subclavian steals occur most frequently on the left side, they are seen on the right occasionally with obstruction of the proximal right subclavian or innominate artery. Most subclavian steals are asymptomatic. When symptoms do occur, the term *subclavian steal syndrome* is used to describe the condition. The symptoms associated with subclavian steal syndrome include dizziness, vertigo, diplopia, ataxia, and bilateral blurred vision. Arm claudication or numbness is not common but may occur in approximately one-third of patients.

- Rumwell C, McPharlin M: *Vascular Technology: An Illustrated Review*, 5th edition. Pasadena, Davies Publishing, 2015, pp 249–250.
- Ku DN, Lumsden A: Blood flow patterns in cerebrovascular disease. In Bernstein EF (ed): *Noninvasive Diagnostic Techniques in Vascular Disease*, 3rd edition. St. Louis, Mosby, 1985, pp 73–83.

Q 65

A complication of plaque ulceration is:

a. thrombosis
b. intraplaque hemorrhage
c. embolization
d. all of the above

A 65

D. All of the above.

Ulceration of an atherosclerotic plaque can be described as erosion of the intimal layer over the plaque surface. This may progress to deep ulceration with embolization of plaque fragments. Thrombus formation is initiated by erosion of the plaque surface. Platelet aggregation occurs, forming a thrombus directly over the ulceration. Distal embolization of thrombus fragments may be the source of transient ischemic attacks (TIAs). Intraplaque hemorrhage can occur as leakage of blood into the atherosclerotic plaque through the ulceration or by rupture of the vasa vasorum.

▸ Rumwell C, McPharlin M: *Vascular Technology: An Illustrated Review*, 5th edition. Pasadena, Davies Publishing, 2015, pp 211–213.

Q 66

A 35-year-old female presents with Horner syndrome and left periorbital headache; she has a history of cystic medial necrosis. Duplex carotid ultrasound reveals two channels of flow within the left common carotid artery separated by a thin echogenic flap. What is the most likely diagnosis?

a. common carotid artery dissection

b. Takayasu's arteritis

c. fibromuscular dysplasia

d. severe stenosis with plaque ulceration

A 66

A. Common carotid artery dissection.

Spontaneous dissection of the cervical carotid arteries most commonly occurs in young patients. Etiologic factors include fibromuscular dysplasia, trauma, cystic medial necrosis, and Marfan syndrome. Initially two channels of flow are present, the true lumen and a false lumen in which the blood flow tunnels between the layers of the vessel wall. This tunneling can create an intimal flap that may be visible sonographically. Dissection can result in thrombosis of the false channel, creating a long, smooth, tapering stenosis. Complete arterial thrombosis may also occur. The clinical presentation usually affects the ipsilateral eye or hemisphere. Headache is present in about 75% of patients. A headache behind the eye is particularly suggestive of ipsilateral carotid dissection.

- Rumwell C, McPharlin M: *Vascular Technology: An Illustrated Review*, 5th edition. Pasadena, Davies Publishing, 2015, pp 52, 215.
- Provenzale JM: Dissection of the internal carotid and vertebral arteries: imaging features. AJR 165:1099–1104, 1995.

Q 67

What is the most common location in the cerebrovascular system for atherosclerosis to occur?

a. intracranial internal carotid artery

b. left subclavian artery

c. innominate artery

d. the carotid bulb

DAVIES
Registry Reviews & Study Aids

A 67

D. The carotid bulb.

Q 68

A 65-year-old male with hypertension and diabetes presents to the vascular lab for cerebrovascular testing due to a right asymptomatic bruit. All of the following could be considered a potential source of the bruit **EXCEPT**:

a. external carotid artery stenosis

b. subclavian artery stenosis

c. common carotid artery occlusion

d. common carotid artery dissection

A 68

C. Common carotid artery occlusion.

A totally occluded vessel will not produce a bruit. A bruit is a result of vibration in the tissue surrounding a stenosis.

▶ Rumwell C, McPharlin M: *Vascular Technology: An Illustrated Review*, 5th edition. Pasadena, Davies Publishing, 2015, p 56.

Q 69

A patient is referred for duplex examination to evaluate a prominent pulsatility felt in the base of the right neck. What is the most likely etiology of this physical finding?

a. excessive CCA tortuosity

b. CCA aneurysm

c. CCA dissection

d. CCA occlusion

A 69

A. Excessive CCA tortuosity.

By far the most common etiology of a pulsatile mass in the base of the neck is excessive tortuosity of the proximal CCA. Although an aneurysm would produce the same physical findings, aneurysms of the carotid artery are quite rare.

Q 70

Of the following, which is **NOT** one of the main collateral pathways in the event of ICA obstruction?

a. genicular to arcuate branches

b. ECA branches to ophthalmic branches

c. contralateral hemisphere

d. posterior to anterior pathways

A 70

A. Genicular to arcuate branches.

Genicular arteries are around the knee; arcuate arteries are in the kidneys.

- Pellerito JS, Polak JF: *Introduction to Vascular Ultrasonography*, 6th edition. Philadelphia, Elsevier Saunders, 2012, pp 111–113, 174–176.
- Pellerito JS, Polak JF: *Introduction to Vascular Ultrasonography*, 7th edition. Philadelphia, Elsevier Saunders, 2020.

Q 71

Your patient undergoes carotid endarterectomy. Six months later angiography is performed because of symptoms referable to the other side. The angiogram reveals that the operated carotid is significantly narrowed. The most likely cause is:

a. atherosclerotic plaque recurrence

b. carotid dissection

c. neointimal hyperplasia

d. embolic activity

A 71

C. Neointimal hyperplasia.

This is a common phenomenon following any trauma to an arterial wall, including endarterectomy and angioplasty. It involves proliferation of smooth-muscle cells in response to the injury.

- Rumwell CB, McPharlin M: *Vascular Technology: An Illustrated Review*, 5th edition. Pasadena, Davies Publishing, 2015, p 216.
- Clowes AW: Pathologic intimal hyperplasia as a response to vascular injury and reconstruction. In Rutherford RB (ed): *Vascular Surgery*, 5th edition. Philadelphia, Saunders, 2000, p 409.

Q 72

A unilateral temporary vision loss associated with cerebrovascular disease is known as:

a. dysphasia

b. amaurosis fugax

c. ataxia

d. diplopia

A 72

B. Amaurosis fugax.

Amaurosis fugax is frequently described by patients as "a shade coming down over one eye." It may be due to an embolic process from the ipsilateral internal carotid artery. The embolus courses from the internal carotid artery to the ophthalmic artery. Other sources of emboli include the common carotid artery and heart.

▸ Rumwell C, McPharlin M: *Vascular Technology: An Illustrated Review*, 5th edition. Pasadena, Davies Publishing, 2015, p 219.

Q 73

Which of the following is a symptom of vertebrobasilar insufficiency?

a. unilateral paresis
b. diplopia
c. aphasia
d. amaurosis fugax

A 73

B. Diplopia.

Diplopia, or double vision, is a symptom of vertebrobasilar insufficiency. Other symptoms of vertebrobasilar insufficiency include numbness around the lips and mouth, poor coordination, dysphagia, vertigo, amnesia, and ataxia.

▶ Rumwell C, McPharlin M: *Vascular Technology: An Illustrated Review*, 5th edition. Pasadena, Davies Publishing, 2015, pp 218–219.

Q 74

A patient presents with right arm numbness and transient loss of vision in the left eye. Which vessel is the most likely source of these symptoms?

a. right external carotid artery

b. right internal carotid artery

c. left internal carotid artery

d. left subclavian artery

A 74

C. Left internal carotid artery.

Unilateral symptoms involving the eye are associated with disease of the ipsilateral internal carotid artery, whereas unilateral symptoms involving the body are associated with the contralateral internal carotid artery.

Q 75

A 56-year-old male presents with transient numbness in the fingers of the left hand. Bilateral brachial systolic blood pressures are 130 mmHg on the right and 105 mmHg on the left. What is the suspected diagnosis?

a. right subclavian artery occlusion

b. innominate artery occlusion

c. left vertebral stenosis

d. left subclavian stenosis

A 75

D. Left subclavian stenosis.

A difference between the brachial blood pressures of 15–20 mmHg suggests subclavian stenosis on the side of the lower pressure.

▶ Rumwell C, McPharlin M: *Vascular Technology: An Illustrated Review*, 5th edition. Pasadena, Davies Publishing, 2015, pp 249–250.

Q 76

Which of the following refers to neurologic symptoms that are of short duration, completely resolving in less than 24 hours?

a. CVA

b. TIA

c. HTN

d. RIND

A 76

B. TIA.

A *reversible ischemic neurologic deficit* (RIND) lasts longer than a *transient ischemic attack* (TIA) but does completely resolve. A *cerebrovascular accident* (CVA) is another term for completed stroke and results in permanent damage.

▸ Rumwell C, McPharlin M: *Vascular Technology: An Illustrated Review*, 5th edition. Pasadena, Davies Publishing, 2015, pp 209–210.

Q 77

A right-handed patient presents with expressive aphasia and left paresis. The cause of these symptoms is most likely obstruction of which of the following vessels?

a. right internal carotid artery
b. left internal carotid artery
c. left vertebral artery
d. basilar artery

A 77

A. Right internal carotid artery.

A lesion in the left middle cerebral artery may cause dysphasia or aphasia. The left hemisphere of the brain controls the right side of the body and vice versa. In a right-handed person, the left hemisphere is dominant for speech. In a left-handed person, the right hemisphere would be dominant, and a lesion in the right middle cerebral artery would produce the symptoms. Paresis (weakness or paralysis) on one side of the body would result from an atherosclerotic lesion in the opposite side.

Q 78

A 57-year-old female presents with numbness in both the right leg and the left arm. These symptoms are most closely associated with:

a. left internal carotid obstruction

b. right internal carotid obstruction

c. vertebrobasilar obstruction

d. right common carotid obstruction

A 78

C. Vertebrobasilar obstruction.

Bilateral symptoms of weakness or numbness are most commonly associated with vertebrobasilar disease. Symptoms of carotid-territory cerebrovascular insufficiency, by contrast, are unilateral. Other vertebrobasilar symptoms include diplopia, bilateral visual blurring, hoarseness, dysarthria, dysphasia, ataxia, and disturbance of equilibrium. Dizziness, vertigo, and drop attacks are not considered symptoms of focal vertebrobasilar disease unless they are associated with other symptoms noted above.

- Rumwell C, McPharlin M: *Vascular Technology: An Illustrated Review*, 5th edition. Pasadena, Davies Publishing, 2015, pp 217–219.

Q 79

What is the name for an abnormal sound caused by flow turbulence and heard on auscultation?

a. thrill

b. bruit

c. Bernoulli

d. Poiseuille

A 79

B. Bruit.

Q 80

What should the patient be asked to do to facilitate auscultation of the carotid artery?

a. breathe regularly and deeply

b. perform the Valsalva maneuver

c. breathe quietly

d. suspend respiration

A 80

D. Suspend respiration.

- Rumwell C, McPharlin M: *Vascular Technology: An Illustrated Review*, 5th edition. Pasadena, Davies Publishing, 2015, p 213.
- Fahey VA: Clinical assessment of the vascular system. In Fahey VA (ed): *Vascular Nursing*, 4th edition. St. Louis, Saunders, 2004, pp 49–71.

Q 81

What are Hollenhorst plaques?

a. cholesterol emboli seen on ophthalmoscopic exam within the retinal artery branches

b. complex plaques in which hemorrhage into necrotic areas has occurred

c. fibrous plaques containing an excessive amount of lipid material

d. ulcerated plaques with thrombus formation

A 81

A. Cholesterol emboli seen on ophthalmoscopic exam within the retinal artery branches.

- Rumwell C, McPharlin M: *Vascular Technology: An Illustrated Review*, 5th edition. Pasadena, Davies Publishing, 2015, p 213.
- Fahey VA: Clinical assessment of the vascular system. In Fahey VA (ed): *Vascular Nursing*, 4th edition. St. Louis, Saunders, 2004, pp 49–71.

Q 82

Neurologic exam of a patient suspected of extracranial cerebrovascular disease should include evaluation of:

a. level of consciousness

b. basic comprehension

c. orientation to time and place

d. all of the above

A 82

D. All of the above.

Q 83

A decreased radial pulse on one arm raises suspicion for:

a. contralateral vertebral stenosis
b. ipsilateral common carotid occlusion
c. ipsilateral subclavian artery stenosis
d. all of the above

A 83

C. Ipsilateral subclavian artery stenosis.

Q 84

What is the purpose of obtaining bilateral blood pressures when evaluating a patient for cerebrovascular disease?

a. The systolic components from each arm are added and the average is calculated to determine the likelihood of cerebrovascular disease.

b. It is necessary to know both brachial pressures to rule out the presence of hypoperfusion syndrome.

c. The brachial blood pressures are compared to see if they are equal.

d. Both brachial blood pressures must be known to determine if hypertension is present.

A 84

C. The brachial blood pressures are compared to see if they are equal.

If one pressure is 15–20 mmHg less than the other, subclavian stenosis or steal is suspected on the side of the lower pressure.

Q 85

Which measurement is most commonly used in angiographic reports of carotid stenosis?

a. percentage area reduction

b. percentage diameter reduction

A 85

B. Percentage diameter reduction.

Percentage diameter reduction is the most common measurement parameter used in angiography as it is easily determined from a longitudinal image. Percentage area reduction is calculated from a cross-sectional image.

▶ Rumwell C, McPharlin M: *Vascular Technology: An Illustrated Review*, 5th edition. Pasadena, Davies Publishing, 2015, pp 253–256.

Q 86

In a symmetric narrowing of the carotid artery, what percentage area reduction most closely corresponds to a percentage diameter reduction of 50%?

a. 75%

b. 90%

c. 50%

d. 35%

A 86

A. 75%.

In a symmetric narrowing, a 50% diameter stenosis is approximately the same as a 75% area stenosis.

- Rumwell C, McPharlin M: *Vascular Technology: An Illustrated Review*, 5th edition. Pasadena, Davies Publishing, 2015, p 256.

Q 87

Percentage diameter and area reduction measurements are most accurate when obtained in which imaging plane?

a. transverse

b. coronal

c. sagittal

d. oblique

A 87

A. Transverse.

Both percentage diameter and percentage area measurements are most accurate when obtained in the transverse scan plane. Percentage stenosis measurements obtained from sagittal or coronal scan planes are easily over- or underestimated because atherosclerotic plaque is typically asymmetric. A sagittal slice obtained through the greatest dimension of asymmetric plaque will overestimate percentage stenosis, whereas a sagittal slice through the smallest dimension of the plaque will underestimate it.

- Ridgway DP: *Introduction to Vascular Scanning: A Guide for the Complete Beginner*, 4th edition. Pasadena, Davies Publishing, 2014, pp 84–86.

Q 88

Which procedure consists of the surgical removal of the atherosclerotic plaque from an artery?

a. atherectomy

b. angioplasty

c. thrombectomy

d. endarterectomy

A 88

D. Endarterectomy.

Q 89

Which diagnostic test most readily differentiates between primary ischemic and primary hemorrhagic stroke?

a. magnetic resonance angiography
b. computed tomography of the brain
c. duplex ultrasonography
d. electrocardiogram

A 89

B. Computed tomography of the brain.

▶ Kelley RE: Stroke prevention and intervention. Postgraduate Medicine 103:43–62, 1998.

Q 90

Which of these statements does **NOT** apply to continuous-wave (CW) Doppler?

a. In CW Doppler range-gating is applied to control vessel selection.

b. The difference between the transmitted and received frequencies falls within the audible hearing range.

c. CW Doppler shows greater spectral broadening than pulsed-wave Doppler.

d. CW Doppler requires both a transmitting and a receiving transducer.

A 90

A. This statement–"In CW Doppler range-gating is applied to control vessel selection"–is **NOT** true.

Range-gating is a method applied to pulsed-wave (not CW) Doppler; it allows signals only from a specified depth to be processed for display. The vascular technologist determines the depth of interest by placement of the sample volume. Because both the speed of sound in tissue (1540 m/sec) and the depth of interest (depth of sample volume) are known, the system can easily calculate the round-trip time of the ultrasound beam from the transducer to the depth of interest and back again, receiving echoes only at that time.

Q 91

In pulsed-wave Doppler studies, loss of the spectral window characterizes which type of blood flow?

a. parabolic flow

b. turbulent flow

c. laminar flow

d. all of the above

A 91

B. Turbulent flow.

The spectral window is the blank, signal-free area underneath systole on the spectral waveform. It is filled in or “lost” when turbulent flow creates spectral broadening. Other reasons for loss of the spectral window include overuse of Doppler gain and incorrect positioning of the sample volume outside of the center streamline (depicting signals from the vessel wall or adjacent slower-moving blood flow).

Q 92

What is indicated by a unilateral decrease in or absence of diastolic flow in the common carotid artery?

a. proximal disease of the aortic arch

b. distal obstructive disease

c. arteriovenous fistula

d. poor cardiac output

A 92

B. Distal obstructive disease.

A unilateral finding of decreased or absent diastolic flow in the common carotid artery is indicative of distal obstructive disease. The most likely scenario is occlusion of the cervical internal carotid artery, although high-grade stenosis of the intracranial internal carotid artery may also produce this finding.

Q 93

This image is a sagittal view of the right vertebral artery origin. Both the subclavian artery and the proximal vertebral artery are demonstrated. The arrow is pointing to what vessel?

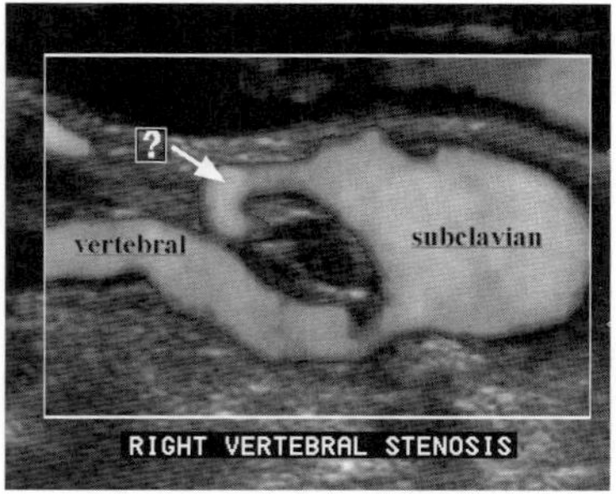

a. inferior thyroid artery

b. ascending pharyngeal artery

c. thyrocervical trunk

d. internal thoracic artery

DAVIES
Registry Reviews & Study Aids

A 93

C. Thyrocervical trunk.

The thyrocervical trunk arises from the subclavian artery near the origin of the vertebral artery. The vertebral artery originates from the posterior aspect of the subclavian artery, whereas the thyrocervical trunk originates from its anterior aspect. The examiner can further differentiate the two vessels by following the vertebral artery into the transverse processes of the cervical spine. The thyrocervical trunk does not enter the spine and will course medially.

Q 94

What frequency is most commonly used for transcranial Doppler?

a. 7.5 MHz

b. 3 MHz

c. 5 MHz

d. 2 MHz

A 94

D. 2 MHz.

A low-frequency transducer is required for transcranial Doppler because the beam must first penetrate the temporal bone. The mean loss of power in penetrating the skull is about 80%. Higher frequencies such as those used for imaging (3–10 MHz) do not provide adequate penetration for insonating the cranial vasculature.

▸ Rumwell C, McPharlin M: *Vascular Technology: An Illustrated Review*, 5th edition. Pasadena, Davies Publishing, 2015, pp 240–242.

Q 95

In conventional transcranial Doppler, the angle of insonation is assumed to be:

a. 0°

b. 45°

c. 60°

d. 90°

A 95

A. 0°.

Because the actual vessel is not visualized with this technique, the angle of incidence is assumed to be zero degrees for calculation of velocities.

- Rumwell C, McPharlin M: *Vascular Technology: An Illustrated Review*, 5th edition. Pasadena, Davies Publishing, 2015, p 240.
- Ridgway DP: *Introduction to Vascular Scanning: A Guide for the Complete Beginner*, 4th edition. Pasadena, Davies Publishing, 2014, p 407.

Q 96

In evaluation of arterial vasospasm following subarachnoid hemorrhage, which testing method would be most useful?

a. CW Doppler

b. OPG-Gee

c. periorbital Doppler

d. transcranial Doppler

A 96

D. Transcranial Doppler.

One of the most widespread applications of transcranial Doppler is the evaluation of the onset, severity, and time course of arterial vasospasm caused by subarachnoid hemorrhage.

▶ Rumwell C, McPharlin M: *Vascular Technology: An Illustrated Review*, 5th edition. Pasadena, Davies Publishing, 2015, pp 244–245.

Q 97

Unilateral increased diastolic flow in the external carotid artery is commonly seen with:

a. external carotid artery stenosis

b. ipsilateral internal carotid artery occlusion

c. ipsilateral common carotid artery occlusion

d. all of the above

A 97

D. All of the above.

The external carotid artery may show increases in both systolic and diastolic flow with stenosis. This can create confusion when both the external and internal carotid arteries are stenotic. Additionally, when the external carotid artery is used as a collateral pathway through the orbit into the intracranial circulation, the diastolic flow will be increased. This can occur with extracranial occlusion of the internal and/or common carotid arteries.

Q 98

The presence of aliasing in the spectral waveform of the internal carotid artery ALWAYS indicates:

a. a hemodynamically significant stenosis of the internal carotid artery
b. an occlusion of the internal carotid artery
c. the frequency shift exceeds ½ the system pulse repetition frequency
d. the wall filter is set too high

A 98

C. The frequency shift exceeds ½ the system pulse repetition frequency (PRF).

The presence or absence of aliasing in the spectral waveform cannot be used as an indicator of disease. Aliasing occurs when the received frequency shift is greater than ½ the system PRF or sampling rate. The frequency shift may be high because of small Doppler angles or high flow velocities. Aliasing may also be seen at steeper angles of incidence and lower velocities when the system PRF is set to a low value.

- Ridgway DP: *Introduction to Vascular Scanning: A Guide for the Complete Beginner*, 4th edition. Pasadena, Davies Publishing, 2014, pp 419–450.

Q 99

The point at which aliasing occurs is known as:

a. Poiseuille's point

b. the Nyquist limit

c. Bernoulli's point

d. the Reynolds number

A 99

B. The Nyquist limit.

Q 100

Which of the following is an appropriate angle for Doppler insonation of the extracranial vasculature?

a. 60°

b. 80°

c. 90°

d. 70°

A 100

A. 60°.

Whenever possible, the Doppler angle of incidence should not exceed 60°. As the angle of incidence exceeds 60°, the accuracy of velocity estimation diminishes. Therefore, Doppler interrogation should be performed only at angles of 60° or less.

- Rumwell CB, McPharlin M: *Vascular Technology: An Illustrated Review*, 5th edition. Pasadena, Davies Publishing, 2015, p 223.
- Ridgway DP: *Introduction to Vascular Scanning: A Guide for the Complete Beginner*, 4th edition. Pasadena, Davies Publishing, 2014, p 426.

Q 101

Which of the following parameters may **NOT** be used to determine the degree of stenosis in the internal carotid artery?

a. heart rate

b. peak frequency shift

c. peak systolic velocity

d. ICA/CCA ratio

A 101

A. Heart rate.

- Ridgway DP: *Introduction to Vascular Scanning: A Guide for the Complete Beginner*, 4th edition. Pasadena, Davies Publishing, 2014, pp 82–90.

Q 102

Which letter in the illustration is pointing to end diastole?

a. A

b. B

c. C

d. D

e. E

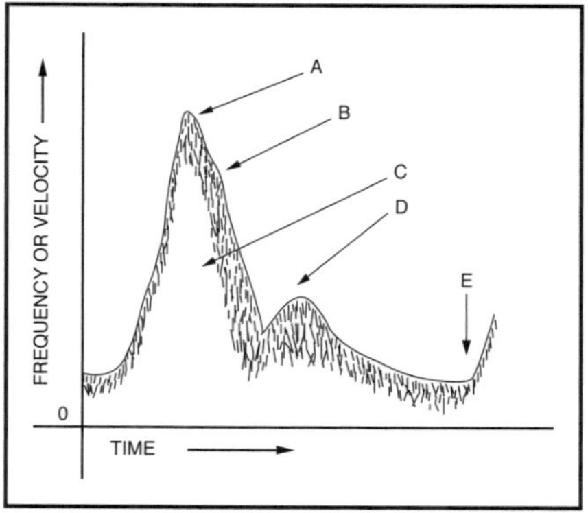

The components of the spectral display.

A 102

E. E.

▸ Ridgway DP: *Introduction to Vascular Scanning: A Guide for the Complete Beginner*, 4th edition. Pasadena, Davies Publishing, 2014, p 80.

Q 103

Which letter represents the spectral window?

a. A

b. B

c. C

d. D

e. E

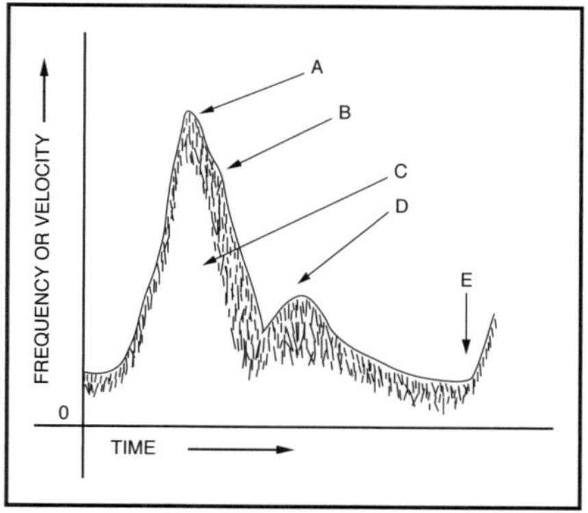

The components of the spectral display.

A 103

C. C.

- Ridgway DP: *Introduction to Vascular Scanning: A Guide for the Complete Beginner*, 4th edition. Pasadena, Davies Publishing, 2014, p 80.

Q 104

Which letter is pointing to the dicrotic notch?

a. A

b. B

c. C

d. D

e. E

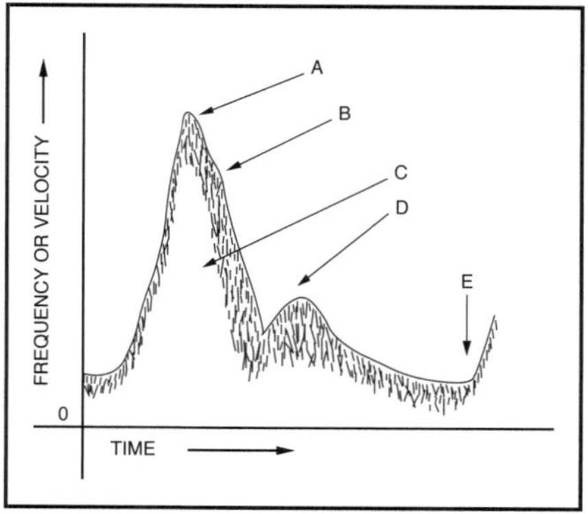

The components of the spectral display.

A 104

D. D.

▶ Ridgway DP: *Introduction to Vascular Scanning: A Guide for the Complete Beginner*, 4th edition. Pasadena, Davies Publishing, 2014, p 80.

Q 105

Which letter is pointing to peak systole?

a. A

b. B

c. C

d. D

e. E

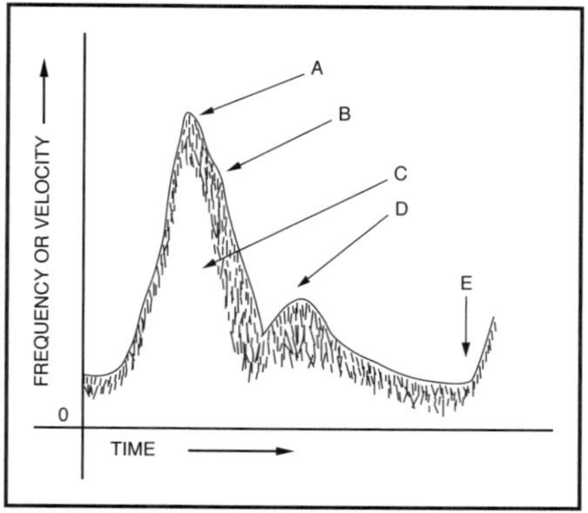

The components of the spectral display.

A 105

A. A.

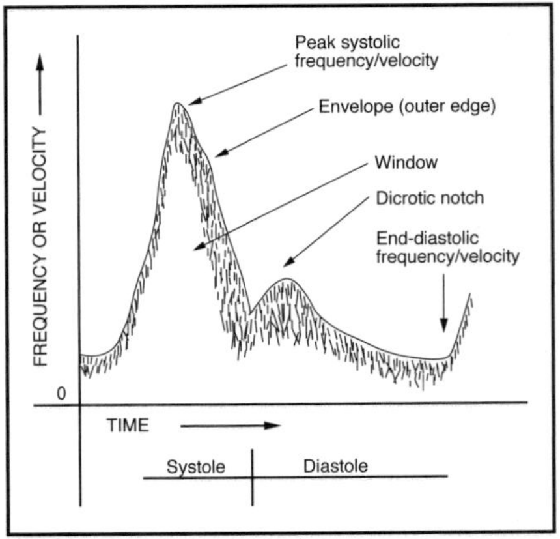

The components of the spectral display.

- Ridgway DP: *Introduction to Vascular Scanning: A Guide for the Complete Beginner*, 4th edition. Pasadena, Davies Publishing, 2014, p 80.

Q 106

Which vessel normally exhibits a triphasic waveform?

a. common carotid artery
b. subclavian artery
c. vertebral artery
d. internal carotid artery

A 106

B. Subclavian artery.

Q 107

On which axis on the spectral display is time displayed?

a. x-axis

b. y-axis

c. z-axis

d. all of the above

A 107

A. x-axis.

Q 108

Which vessel normally supplies blood flow to the face and scalp?

a. internal carotid artery
b. subclavian artery
c. external carotid artery
d. thyrocervical trunk

A 108

C. External carotid artery.

Q 109

On the spectral display, which artery will demonstrate the most prominent oscillations in response to manual tapping on the superficial temporal artery?

a. thyrocervical trunk

b. external carotid artery

c. subclavian artery

d. internal carotid artery

A 109

B. External carotid artery.

The “temporal tap” has been a widely taught method of distinguishing the ECA from the ICA and CCA. In clinical practice, however, the author has not found the temporal tap to be a useful technique for localizing the external carotid artery. Oscillations are frequently seen in the ICA and CCA that are as strong as or stronger than those seen in the ECA. It is better to differentiate the ICA and ECA by evaluating waveform characteristics, vessel positions, and the presence of branches. In a study published in *Radiology* in 1996, Kliewer et al. found that “the temporal tap alone may not reliably distinguish the ECA from the ICA or CCA.”

▸ Kliewer MA, Freed KS, Hertzberg BS, et al: Temporal artery tap. Radiology 201:481–484, 1996.

Q 110

What term describes this waveform?

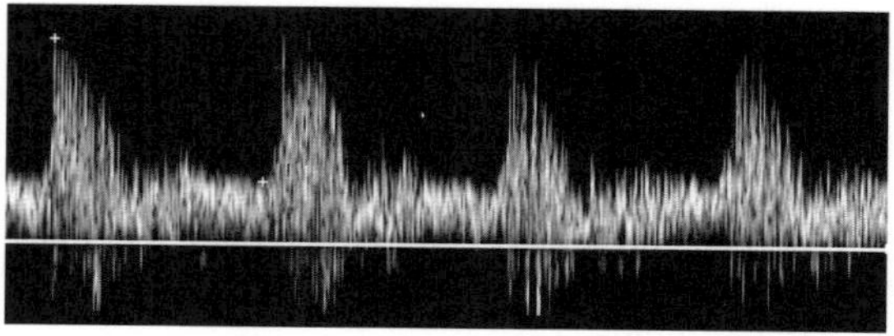

a. tardus parvus
b. high resistance
c. dampened
d. spectral broadening

A 110

D. Spectral broadening.

On this waveform, the spectral window is "lost" or filled in. Spectral broadening represents the reflection of a wide range of frequency shifts due to interaction of the Doppler beam with a wide range of flow velocities, as in poststenotic turbulence. Spectral broadening can be thought of as a broadening of the returning spectrum of frequencies.

▸ Rumwell C, McPharlin M: *Vascular Technology: An Illustrated Review*, 5th edition. Pasadena, Davies Publishing, 2015, pp 57–68.

Q 111

What type of occlusion is indicated when transcranial Doppler detects an abnormal flow direction in the left anterior cerebral artery?

a. right internal carotid artery occlusion

b. left internal carotid artery occlusion

c. right vertebral artery occlusion

d. left external carotid artery occlusion

A 111

B. Left internal carotid artery occlusion.

Crossover collateralization may occur from one anterior cerebral artery through the anterior communicating artery to the contralateral anterior cerebral artery in cases of internal carotid artery occlusion on the same side as the reversed flow. For example, if the left internal carotid artery is occluded, the left middle cerebral artery may be supplied by reversed flow in the ipsilateral (left) anterior cerebral artery. The left anterior cerebral artery will receive its flow from the right anterior cerebral artery via the anterior communicating artery.

▶ Rumwell C, McPharlin M: *Vascular Technology: An Illustrated Review*, 5th edition. Pasadena, Davies Publishing, 2015, p 243.

Q 112

Waveforms obtained from an artery supplying an intracranial arteriovenous malformation will exhibit:

a. absent diastolic flow

b. decreased velocities

c. triphasic flow

d. a low pulsatility index

A 112

D. A low pulsatility index.

An artery that feeds an arteriovenous malformation will show increased velocities in both systole and diastole. The diastolic velocity especially will be increased, resulting in a waveform with very low resistance. A waveform that exhibits low resistance will have a low pulsatility index and low resistive index measurement.

▸ Rumwell C, McPharlin M: *Vascular Technology: An Illustrated Review*, 5th edition. Pasadena, Davies Publishing, 2015, pp 246–247.

Q 113

During a transcranial Doppler study, with the probe placed over the right temporal bone, how will flow in the right anterior cerebral artery be oriented?

a. The right middle cerebral artery cannot be seen from this window.
b. toward the probe
c. at 90° to the probe
d. away from the probe

A 113

D. Away from the probe.

Q 114

In transcranial Doppler studies, which vessel is evaluated from the foramen magnum window?

a. posterior communicating artery

b. anterior communicating artery

c. basilar artery

d. posterior cerebral artery

A 114

C. Basilar artery.

For the transforaminal (suboccipital) window, the probe is placed at the foramen magnum with the transducer angled superiorly toward the eyes. From this view, signals can be obtained from the intracranial portion of both vertebral arteries as well as the basilar artery.

- Rumwell C, McPharlin M: *Vascular Technology: An Illustrated Review*, 5th edition. Pasadena, Davies Publishing, 2015, p 242.
- Tegeler CH, Eicke M: Physics and principles of transcranial Doppler ultrasonography. In Babikian VL (ed): *Transcranial Doppler Ultrasonography*. St. Louis, Mosby, 1993.

Q 115

In transcranial Doppler, with the probe placed at the foramen magnum window, flow toward the probe in the vertebral artery is indicative of:

a. normality

b. basilar artery stenosis

c. subclavian steal

d. internal carotid stenosis

A 115

C. Subclavian steal.

With the probe placed at the foramen magnum window, flow in the intracranial vertebral arteries moves away from the probe, demonstrating the retrograde flow characteristic of subclavian steal. This results in a negative Doppler shift.

- Rumwell C, McPharlin M: *Vascular Technology: An Illustrated Review*, 5th edition. Pasadena, Davies Publishing, 2015, pp 249–251.
- Tegeler CH, Eicke M: Physics and principles of transcranial Doppler ultrasonography. In Babikian VL (ed): *Transcranial Doppler Ultrasonography*. St. Louis, Mosby, 1993.

Q 116

These waveforms were obtained from a 72-year-old asymptomatic male who was referred for duplex carotid ultrasound prior to undergoing surgery. The waveform at top is of the left common carotid artery. The waveform at bottom is of the right common carotid artery. Considering these findings, which of the following diagnoses is most likely?

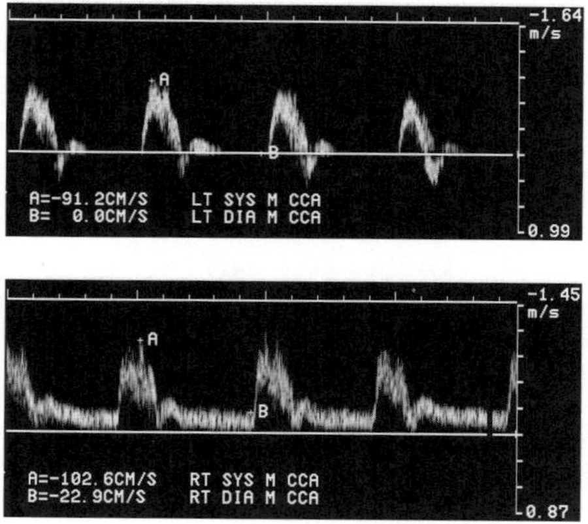

a. left arteriovenous fistula
b. left internal carotid occlusion
c. right common carotid stenosis
d. right innominate occlusion

A 116

B. Left internal carotid occlusion.

Comparison of both common carotid artery waveforms is an important aspect of a duplex carotid study. Both sides should show a similar amount of diastolic flow. A unilateral decrease in diastole should increase suspicion for distal occlusive disease on the ipsilateral side. In other words, if the left common carotid artery shows decreased diastolic flow, distal occlusive disease involving the left internal carotid artery is suspected. Most commonly, the disease is present in the extracranial portion of the internal carotid artery near the origin, although if this portion of the internal carotid artery is normal, significant stenosis or occlusion should be suspected in the intracranial portion of the same internal carotid artery at the level of the siphon.

Q 117

What is most likely indicated by the presence of a mosaic pattern in the color Doppler image of the internal carotid artery?

a. reversed flow in the vertebral artery

b. slow flow proximal to an occlusion

c. the presence of poststenotic turbulence

d. improper color setup with the pulse repetition frequency set too high

A 117

C. The presence of poststenotic turbulence.

A mosaic pattern on color Doppler imaging results from the reflection of a wide range of frequency shifts back to the transducer. The most likely reason for this is the wide range of velocities and flow directions present in poststenotic turbulence. Spectral broadening results in the display of a multitude of colors. Some of the colors represent aliasing caused by the higher velocities present in the poststenotic turbulence. Other colors represent reversed flow in the eddies seen distal to stenoses. The mosaic pattern alerts the examiner to the likelihood of high-grade stenosis. A similar appearance may be seen with color Doppler aliasing when the pulse repetition frequency is set too low for the type of flow being evaluated. In this situation, however, the angle-corrected Doppler waveform will not reveal increased velocities or spectral broadening.

Q 118

To increase the color Doppler sensitivity when the vessel under interrogation does **NOT** fill well with color, what adjustments should you make in the technical parameters?

a. decrease color pulse repetition frequency, increase color gain, increase color filter

b. increase color pulse repetition frequency, decrease color gain, increase color filter

c. increase color pulse repetition frequency, decrease color gain, decrease color filter

d. decrease color pulse repetition frequency, increase color gain, decrease color filter

A 118

D. Decrease color pulse repetition frequency (PRF), increase color gain, decrease color filter.

When the color Doppler does not fill a vessel as expected, the system parameters should be adjusted to sensitize the color for detection of slow flow. This must be done to rule out the presence of very slow or trickle flow within a vessel. Decreasing the system PRF improves sensitivity to slow flow by increasing the time between transmitted pulses. The greater the time between pulses, the slower the flow that can be detected by the color Doppler. Increasing the color gain improves sensitivity simply by amplifying the returning echoes–similar to the volume control on a radio. Decreasing the color filter increases sensitivity because slow flow produces low-frequency shifts that are eliminated by high wall filter settings. As the color filter is decreased, lower-frequency shifts can pass through the system and be displayed on the color monitor. Unfortunately, as the color filter is lowered, low-frequency shifts from the moving vessel wall and flash artifact from patient breathing or movement are also more likely to be displayed on the color monitor and may partially obscure the vessel.

▸ Ridgway DP: *Introduction to Vascular Scanning: A Guide for the Complete Beginner*, 4th edition. Pasadena, Davies Publishing, 2014, pp 365–370.

Q 119

Which component of the reflected signals does power Doppler encode?

a. amplitude
b. velocity
c. frequency shift
d. wavelength

A 119

A. Amplitude.

Power Doppler colorizes the amplitude of the moving signals. Amplitude depends on the relative number of red blood cells passing through the beam at any given point in time. The brighter the color with power Doppler, the greater the concentration of red blood cells. The dimmer the color, the lower the concentration of red blood cells. Since the frequency shift is not displayed, power Doppler does not show flow direction or as much angle dependence as color Doppler.

Q 120

In this B-mode picture the arrow is pointing to a dark area in the image. What explains this dark area?

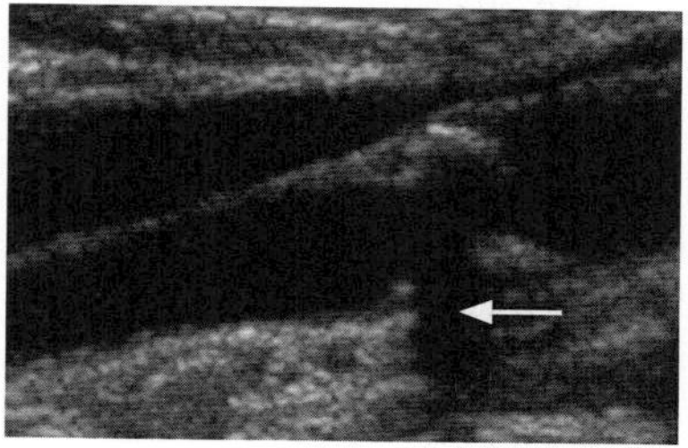

a. shadowing from calcified plaque

b. inadequate amount of gel between transducer face and skin

c. ulcerated plaque

d. bad transducer element

Cerebrovascular / Testing and Treatment / AIT—Hotspot

A 120

A. Shadowing from calcified plaque.

Q 121

This waveform was most likely obtained from which vessel?

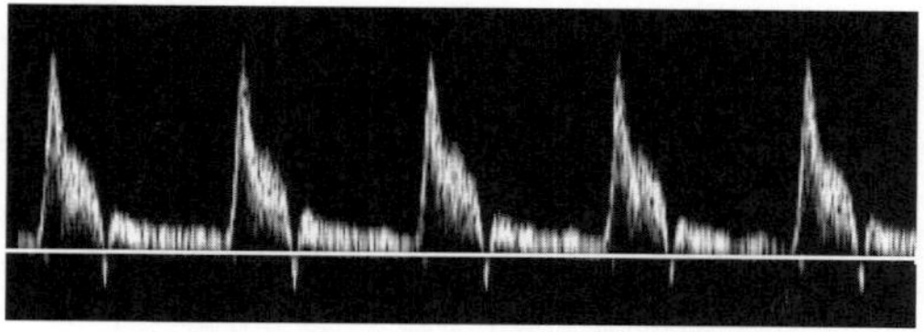

a. vertebral artery

b. internal carotid artery

c. common carotid artery

d. external carotid artery

A 121

D. External carotid artery.

▶ Rumwell C, McPharlin M: *Vascular Technology: An Illustrated Review*, 5th edition. Pasadena, Davies Publishing, 2015, pp 57–68.

Q 122

This waveform can be described as:

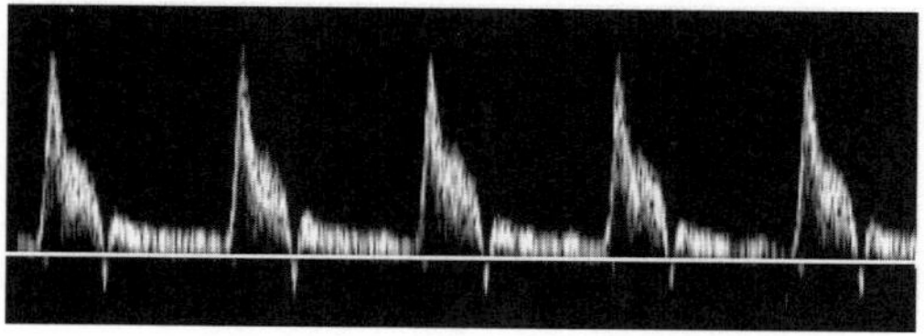

a. monophasic

b. high-resistance

c. low-resistance

d. biphasic

A 122

B. High-resistance.

- Rumwell C, McPharlin M: *Vascular Technology: An Illustrated Review*, 5th edition. Pasadena, Davies Publishing, 2015, pp 57–68.

Q 123

All of the following are consistent with the diagnosis of right internal carotid artery occlusion **EXCEPT**:

a. hyperemic flow in the left common carotid artery
b. increased diastolic flow in the ipsilateral common carotid artery
c. low-resistance flow in the right external carotid artery
d. debris-filled right internal carotid artery

A 123

B. Increased diastolic flow in the ipsilateral common carotid artery is **NOT** a finding associated with right internal carotid artery occlusion.

Findings that may be associated with occlusion of the internal carotid artery include:

1. decreased or absent diastolic flow in the ipsilateral common carotid artery
2. compensatory hyperemic flow in the contralateral common carotid artery
3. increased diastolic flow in the ipsilateral external carotid artery when external-to-internal collateralization occurs through the orbit
4. debris-filled internal carotid artery
5. absence of color fill within the affected internal carotid artery when the system has been sensitized to detect slow flow
6. absence of a spectral Doppler signal within the affected internal carotid artery with the sample volume size opened to include the entire width of the vessel
7. lack of normal pulsatility visible by B-mode in the affected internal carotid artery (a radial "jerking" motion may be detected instead)

Q 124

Duplex findings in a 58-year-old male include a systolic velocity of 58 cm/sec in the right common carotid artery and a systolic velocity of 92 cm/sec in the left common carotid artery. All of the following could contribute to this finding **EXCEPT**:

a. The Doppler angle of incidence was underestimated on the right common carotid artery.

b. There is occlusion of the right internal carotid artery.

c. The Doppler angle of incidence was underestimated on the left common carotid artery.

d. There is occlusion of the innominate artery.

DAVIES
Registry Reviews & Study Aids

A 124

C. The Doppler angle of incidence was underestimated on the left common carotid artery.

Probably the most common error in performance of a duplex ultrasound study is improper measurement of the Doppler angle of incidence. When proper measurement is performed, the angle-correct cursor is aligned parallel to the vessel wall at the point of Doppler sampling. The resultant angle should be 60° or less. If the angle of incidence exceeds 60°, the velocity estimation may be inaccurate. Similarly, if the angle-correct cursor is incorrectly aligned, the velocity estimation will be inaccurate. Overestimation of the angle of incidence will result in overestimation of the velocity, and underestimation of the angle of incidence will result in underestimation of the velocity.

Q 125

This waveform was obtained in the proximal left internal carotid artery of a 62-year-old male. What is the most likely explanation?

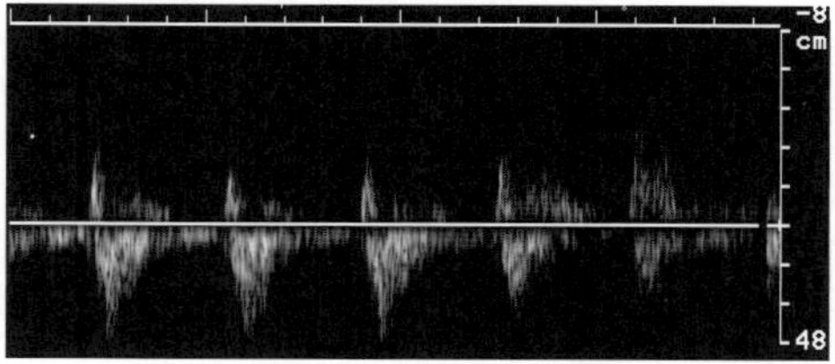

a. reversed flow in a stump proximal to internal carotid artery occlusion

b. reversed internal carotid artery flow due to ipsilateral external carotid artery occlusion

c. improper setup of the system pulse repetition frequency

d. reversed flow in the internal carotid artery due to ipsilateral vertebral artery occlusion

A 125

A. Reversed flow in a stump proximal to internal carotid artery occlusion.

Q 126

The top waveform was obtained from the mid left internal carotid artery and the bottom waveform from the mid right internal carotid artery. What is the most likely diagnosis?

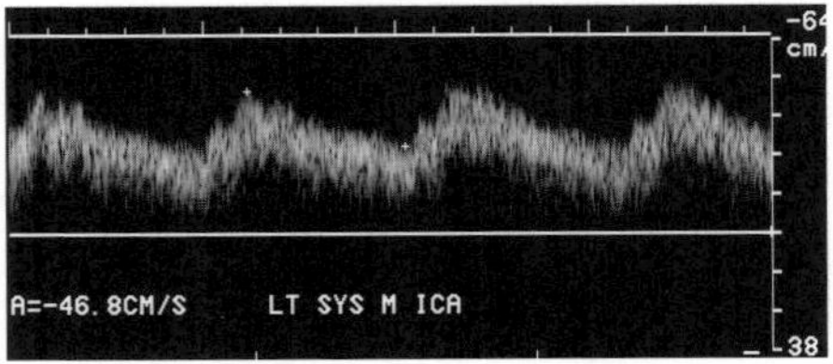

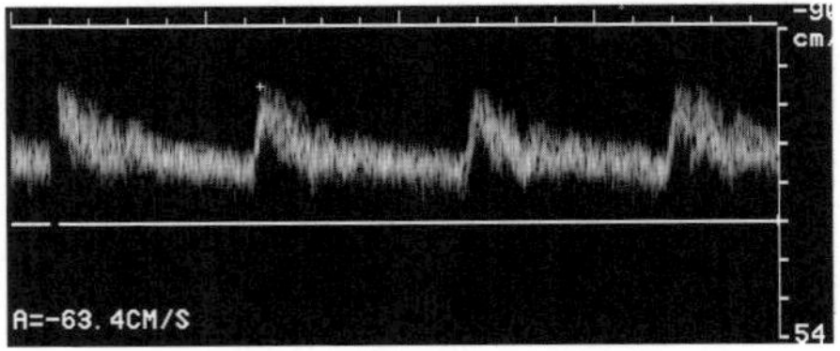

a. distal stenosis in the left internal carotid artery

b. distal stenosis in the right internal carotid artery

c. innominate occlusion

d. high-grade stenosis of the proximal left common carotid artery

A 126

D. High-grade stenosis of the proximal left common carotid artery.

With significant proximal stenosis, the waveforms obtained distal to the disease may show dampening of the systolic component with a delayed systolic rise time. With significant disease distal to the site of sampling, the diastolic component will be dampened because of the increased resistance to flow toward the obstruction.

Q 127

What term can be used to describe this waveform?

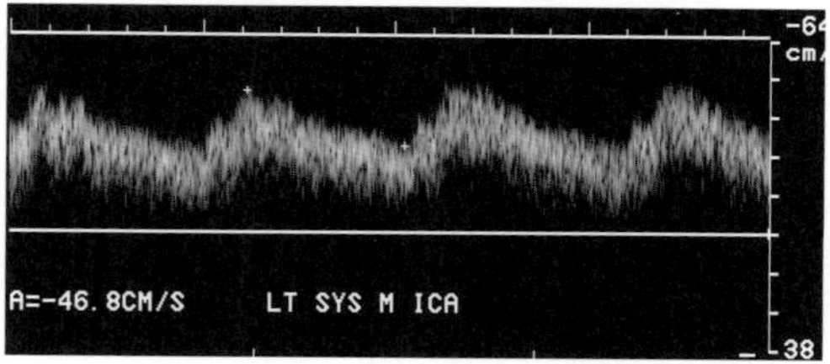

a. high-resistance

b. tardus parvus

c. spectral broadening

d. triphasic

A 127

B. Tardus parvus.

See the answer to question 303.

▶ Rumwell C, McPharlin M: *Vascular Technology: An Illustrated Review*, 5th edition. Pasadena, Davies Publishing, 2015, p 148.

Q 128

Overestimation of the degree of stenosis in the internal carotid artery will **NOT** be due to:

a. increased velocities contralateral to an occlusion

b. improper location of the sample volume proximal to the stenosis

c. vessel tortuosity

d. overestimation of the angle of incidence

A 128

B. Improper location of the sample volume proximal to the stenosis.

Doppler samples obtained proximal to the point of stenosis will produce lower velocities than those obtained at the narrowing, resulting in underestimation, not overestimation, of the degree of stenosis. Overestimation of the Doppler angle will result in overestimation of the velocity. Vessel tortuosities may result in overestimation or underestimation of stenosis because accurate measurement of the Doppler angle is difficult. Velocities contralateral to occlusion may be increased due to compensatory flow. Thus, stenosis is likely to be overestimated when it occurs contralateral to an occlusion.

▶ Rumwell C, McPharlin M: *Vascular Technology: An Illustrated Review*, 5th edition. Pasadena, Davies Publishing, 2015, pp 221–238.

Q 129

An angiogram shows an embolus lodged in the right middle cerebral artery. The source of the embolus could be:

a. nonvalvular atrial fibrillation

b. ulcerated plaque in the right internal carotid artery

c. complex plaque in the right external carotid artery

d. a and b only

A 129

D. A and B only.

The external carotid artery does not feed into the middle cerebral artery, and so complex plaque at this site cannot be a source of emboli for that artery. Ulcerated plaque in the ipsilateral internal or common carotid artery may produce emboli that travel into the middle cerebral artery. Cardiac disease also poses a risk for embolic stroke: Nonvalvular atrial fibrillation and vegetations on valves, among other things, can produce emboli.

▶ Rumwell C, McPharlin M: *Vascular Technology: An Illustrated Review*, 5th edition. Pasadena, Davies Publishing, 2015, pp 199–201.

Q 130

The most commonly used artery for catheter insertion to perform arteriography of the carotid circulation is the:

a. superficial femoral artery

b. axillary artery

c. common femoral artery

d. brachial artery

A 130

C. Common femoral artery.

Q 131

All of the following can be determined from an arteriogram **EXCEPT**:

a. percent diameter stenosis

b. reversed flow in the vertebral

c. flow turbulence

d. arterial dissection

A 131

C. Flow turbulence.

Arteriography shows a two-dimensional view of the anatomy from which percentage diameter stenosis can be measured. Reversed flow can be detected with delayed films, and dissection can be seen as well. Since hemodynamics cannot be evaluated with this technique, flow turbulence is not detected.

Q 132

A duplex image of the carotid bifurcation that demonstrates a goblet-like configuration of the internal and external branches curving around a highly vascularized mass suggests:

a. carotid body tumor

b. severe ICA stenosis

c. temporal arteritis

d. carotid aneurysm

A 132

A. Carotid body tumor.

- Rumwell CB, McPharlin M: *Vascular Technology: An Illustrated Review*, 5th edition. Pasadena, Davies Publishing, 2015, p 214.
- Pellerito JS, Polak JF: *Introduction to Vascular Ultrasonography*, 6th edition. Philadelphia, Elsevier Saunders, 2012, pp 181–183.
- Pellerito JS, Polak JF: *Introduction to Vascular Ultrasonography*, 7th edition. Philadelphia, Elsevier Saunders, 2020.

Q 133

Among the chief limitations of continuous-wave Doppler is/are:

a. Polarity of the reflected signal frequency shift cannot be determined; direction of blood flow cannot be defined.
b. The two-transducer system is inherently more expensive.
c. Depth information is not possible; precise location of flow pattern cannot be determined.
d. The sample volume is too small to interrogate deeper vessels.

A 133

C. Depth information is not possible; precise location of flow pattern cannot be determined.

The two-transducer probes for continuous-wave (CW) Doppler are relatively inexpensive. Directionality is included in most diagnostic-grade CW Doppler systems, and they can be connected to a spectrum analyzer. CW has no sample volume as pulsed Doppler does.

- Pellerito JS, Polak JF: *Introduction to Vascular Ultrasonography*, 6th edition. Philadelphia, Elsevier Saunders, 2012, pp 38–39.
- Pellerito JS, Polak JF: *Introduction to Vascular Ultrasonography*, 7th edition. Philadelphia, Elsevier Saunders, 2020.

Q 134

You perform a transcranial Doppler exam, insonating the left anterior cerebral artery of your patient. The flow is toward the beam. This finding suggests:

a. contralateral carotid obstruction, with left-to-right collateralization
b. ipsilateral carotid obstruction, with posterior-to-anterior collateralization
c. ipsilateral carotid obstruction, with right-to-left collateralization
d. contralateral siphon disease

A 134

C. Ipsilateral carotid obstruction, with right-to-left collateralization.

Flow in the ACA is normally away from the beam, so this is not normal. It suggests flow coming across from the other hemisphere via the anterior communicating artery.

- Pellerito JS, Polak JF: *Introduction to Vascular Ultrasonography*, 6th edition. Philadelphia, Elsevier Saunders, 2012, p 218.
- Pellerito JS, Polak JF: *Introduction to Vascular Ultrasonography*, 7th edition. Philadelphia, Elsevier Saunders, 2020.

Q 135

Following carotid endarterectomy, which of these defects may be visualized with B-mode imaging?

a. intimal flap

b. stricture of the suture line

c. platelet aggregation

d. all of the above

A 135

D. All of the above.

▶ Rumwell C, McPharlin M: *Vascular Technology: An Illustrated Review*, 5th edition. Pasadena, Davies Publishing, 2015, p 237.

Q 136

Blood flow from the deep venous system will back up into the superficial system when:

a. perforating veins are competent
b. perforating veins are incompetent
c. the calf muscles contract
d. normal venous hemodynamics are present

A 136

B. Perforating veins are incompetent.

With incompetent perforating veins, blood will flow retrograde from the deep venous system into the superficial venous system, increasing superficial venous pressure.

▸ Rumwell C, McPharlin M: *Vascular Technology: An Illustrated Review*, 5th edition. Pasadena, Davies Publishing, 2015, p 287.

Q 137

Elevated peripheral venous pressure results in:

a. decreased arterial resis tance

b. edema

c. lymphangitis

d. dependent rubor

A 137

B. Edema.

Q 138

The greatest clinical danger from venous thrombosis is:

a. superficial venous obstruction
b. venous hypertension
c. pulmonary embolism
d. incompetent valves

A 138

C. Pulmonary embolism.

Q 139

Virchow's triad consists of three factors that are significant in the development of venous thrombosis. These are:

a. stasis, hypercoagulability, extrinsic compression
b. hypercoagulability, cancer, stasis
c. stasis, extrinsic compression, trauma
d. trauma, stasis, hypercoagulability

A 139

D. Trauma, stasis, hypercoagulability.

Q 140

What is the most common place for thrombus to begin in the lower extremity?

a. soleal sinuses

b. proximal paratibial perforators (Boyd's veins)

c. femoral canal perforators (Dodd's veins)

d. perforating veins

A 140

A. Soleal sinuses.

In the lower extremity, the soleal sinuses of the calf muscle are the most common site of thrombus formation. See also the answer to question 173.

Q 141

Which of the following is **NOT** a predisposing factor for the development of venous thrombosis?

a. bone fracture
b. pregnancy
c. daily use of aspirin
d. a long airplane trip

A 141

C. Daily use of aspirin.

Pregnancy, bone fracture, or a long airplane trip all can lead to stasis, which is one of the factors in Virchow's triad of factors leading to venous thrombosis.

Q 142

Which statement is **TRUE** regarding incompetent venous valves?

a. Incompetent valves promote flow toward the heart.
b. Incompetent valves result in decreased venous pressure.
c. Incompetent valves may lead to hemosiderin deposition.
d. Incompetent valves decrease the likelihood of venous thrombosis.

DAVIES
Registry Reviews & Study Aids

A 142

C. Incompetent valves may lead to hemosiderin deposition.

Incompetent venous valves may result in increased venous pressure as blood flows retrograde (away from the heart). This produces stasis and the increased likelihood of the development of venous thrombosis. Red blood cells and fibrinogen may leak into the surrounding tissue, leading to hemosiderin deposition. This causes the brawny skin changes that are associated with chronic venous disease.

- Oliver MA: Clinical evaluation. In Talbot SR, Oliver MA: *Techniques of Venous Imaging*. Pasadena, Davies Publishing, 1992, pp 27–36.
- Rumwell C, McPharlin M: *Vascular Technology: An Illustrated Review*, 5th edition. Pasadena, Davies Publishing, 2015, p 287.

Q 143

The most common cause of upper extremity venous thrombus is:

a. intravenous catheters and lines

b. blunt trauma

c. weightlifting

d. pregnancy

A 143

A. Intravenous catheters and lines.

Upper extremity venous thrombosis, once rare, has become much more common due to increased use of intravenous lines and catheters during hospital stays.

Q 144

Primary varicose veins form as a result of:

a. Baker's cysts

b. lymphedema

c. incompetent or absent venous valves

d. venous ulcers

A 144

C. Incompetent or absent venous valves.

Q 145

Lymphedema is a result of:

a. impaired transport of lymph

b. chronic venous insufficiency

c. deep venous thrombosis

d. incompetent venous valves

A 145

A. Impaired transport of lymph.

There is much that is not understood about the etiology of lymphedema. Although clinically it is easily confused with venous thrombosis because of the associated limb swelling, lymphedema is the result of the impaired transport of lymph. This impairment may be caused by a malfunction of lymph nodes, too few lymph nodes, obstructed lymph node pathways, or fluid overload.

- Rumwell C, McPharlin M: *Vascular Technology: An Illustrated Review*, 5th edition. Pasadena, Davies Publishing, 2015, pp 289–292.
- Felty CL, Rooke TW: Lymphedema. In Fahey VA (ed): *Vascular Nursing*, 4th edition. St. Louis, Saunders, 2004.

Q 146

Which statement is **NOT** true regarding varicose veins?

a. Primary varicose veins occur in the great and small saphenous system.
b. Secondary varicose veins result from obstruction of the deep venous system.
c. Secondary varicose veins are the most common type of varicose veins.
d. Stasis in dilated, tortuous varicose veins can lead to thrombosis.

DAVIES Registry Reviews & Study Aids

A 146

C. This statement–"secondary varicose veins are the most common type of varicose veins"–is **NOT** true.

Primary varicose veins are the most common type of varicose veins.

- Rumwell C, McPharlin M: *Vascular Technology: An Illustrated Review*, 5th edition. Pasadena, Davies Publishing, 2015, pp 288–289.
- Kerr KA, Watson WC, Dalsing MC: Chronic venous disease. In Fahey VA (ed): *Vascular Nursing*, 4th edition. St. Louis, Saunders, 2004.

Q 147

Phlegmasia cerulea dolens is a serious condition associated with:

a. cyanosis

b. iliofemoral deep venous thrombosis

c. decreased arterial inflow due to severely reduced venous outflow

d. all of the above

DAVIES
Registry Reviews & Study Aids

A 147

D. All of the above.

▶ Rumwell C, McPharlin M: *Vascular Technology: An Illustrated Review*, 5th edition. Pasadena, Davies Publishing, 2015, p 290.

Q 148

What are the most common features of symptomatic venous thrombosis?

a. Homan's sign
b. ulceration
c. discoloration
d. pain and tenderness

A 148

D. Pain and tenderness.

- Oliver MA: Clinical evaluation. In Talbot SR, Oliver MA: *Techniques of Venous Imaging*. Pasadena, Davies Publishing, 1992, pp 27–36.
- Rumwell C, McPharlin M: *Vascular Technology: An Illustrated Review*, 5th edition. Pasadena, Davies Publishing, 2015, pp 283–284.

Q 149

Which of the following is **NOT** a symptom of pulmonary embolism?

a. claudication

b. dyspnea

c. chest pain

d. tachycardia

A 149

A. Claudication.

A venous thrombus that has embolized to the lungs is known as a pulmonary embolus. Pulmonary embolism may be symptomatic or asymptomatic and is potentially fatal. Symptoms of pulmonary embolism include chest pain, dyspnea, tachycardia, and tachypnea. Claudication is ischemic muscle pain brought on by exercise and relieved by rest.

- Oliver MA: Clinical evaluation. In Talbot SR, Oliver MA: *Techniques of Venous Imaging*. Pasadena, Davies Publishing, 1992, pp 27–36.
- Rumwell C, McPharlin M: *Vascular Technology: An Illustrated Review*, 5th edition. Pasadena, Davies Publishing, 2015, pp 45–46.

Q 150

What is Homan's sign?

a. a highly specific sign for lower extremity venous thrombosis
b. calf discomfort on passive dorsiflexion
c. a highly specific sign for upper extremity venous thrombosis
d. numbness of the digits with hyperextension of an extremity

A 150

B. Calf discomfort on passive dorsiflexion.

Homan's sign is a nonspecific and insensitive sign for venous thrombosis and should not be used.

- Oliver MA: Clinical evaluation. In Talbot SR, Oliver MA: *Techniques of Venous Imaging*. Pasadena, Davies Publishing, 1992, pp 27–36.
- Rumwell C, McPharlin M: *Vascular Technology: An Illustrated Review*, 5th edition. Pasadena, Davies Publishing, 2015, pp 283–284.

Q 151

Which of the following is a sign of chronic venous insufficiency?

a. dyspnea

b. shooting pains in the extremity

c. numbness

d. hyperpigmentation

A 151

D. Hyperpigmentation.

Hyperpigmentation occurs as a result of the breakdown of red blood cells into hemosiderin deposits. (See also the answer to question 142.) Shooting pains are a more common symptom of neuromuscular problems. Dyspnea is a symptom of pulmonary embolism, which is more common in acute cases of venous thrombosis. Numbness is more commonly associated with arterial insufficiency.

▸ Rumwell C, McPharlin M: *Vascular Technology: An Illustrated Review*, 5th edition. Pasadena, Davies Publishing, 2015, pp 284–285.

Q 152

Iliac vein thrombosis most likely results in:

a. no swelling of either extremity
b. unilateral swelling isolated to the calf
c. bilateral calf vein swelling
d. unilateral swelling of the entire lower extremity

A 152

D. Unilateral swelling of the entire lower extremity.

▸ Fahey VA: Clinical assessment of the vascular system. In Fahey VA (ed): *Vascular Nursing*, 4th edition. St. Louis, Saunders, 2004, pp 49–71.

Q 153

Inferior vena cava thrombosis most likely results in:

a. swelling of the right lower extremity only
b. bilateral swelling of the lower extremities
c. unilateral calf vein swelling
d. abdominal cavity swelling

A 153

B. Bilateral swelling of the lower extremities.

Q 154

A 42-year-old female presents with a gradual onset of asymptomatic right lower extremity swelling, which began at the dorsum of the foot and gradually included the whole leg. These findings are most likely associated with:

a. acute deep venous thrombosis involving the popliteal vein

b. Baker's cyst

c. acute superficial venous thrombosis involving the great saphenous vein

d. lymphedema

A 154

D. Lymphedema.

Lymphedema may be very difficult to differentiate from deep venous thrombosis clinically. The gradual onset of swelling over a period of several months, which begins at the dorsum of the foot and is not associated with other symptoms, is characteristic of lymphedema. Acute DVT involving the popliteal vein would produce swelling in the calf associated with pain or tenderness that was not of a gradual onset. Superficial venous thrombosis of the great saphenous vein would most likely produce pain and tenderness over the thrombus site. A Baker's cyst will not cause swelling of the entire lower extremity.

- Rumwell C, McPharlin M: *Vascular Technology: An Illustrated Review*, 5th edition. Pasadena, Davies Publishing, 2015, pp 288–292.
- Felty CL, Rooke TW: Lymphedema. In Fahey VA (ed): *Vascular Nursing*, 4th edition. St. Louis, Saunders, 2004.

Q 155

Which finding is **NOT** associated with venous ulcers?

a. shiny skin

b. location near medial malleolus

c. irregular borders

d. brawny discoloration

A 155

A. Shiny skin is **NOT** associated with venous ulcers.

Venous ulcers tend to have a brawny discoloration. Arterial ulcers exhibit shiny skin with loss of hair.

▶ Rumwell C, McPharlin M: *Vascular Technology: An Illustrated Review*, 5th edition. Pasadena, Davies Publishing, 2015, pp 55, 289–290.

Q 156

The most important technique in physical examination of the venous system is:

a. auscultation

b. inspection

c. palpation

d. a and c

A 156

B. Inspection.

Because venous sounds are not audible with a stethoscope, auscultation is not helpful except in cases of arteriovenous fistula. Palpation offers only minimal information in evaluation of the venous system. Inspection of the extremities, however, is very important. The patient suspected of venous disease is inspected for limb swelling, ulceration, color changes, and cellulitis.

▸ Rumwell C, McPharlin M: *Vascular Technology: An Illustrated Review*, 5th edition. Pasadena, Davies Publishing, 2015, pp 288–292.

Q 157

What is the term for persistent inflammation of the skin around the ankle with a tendency toward a brown pigmentation?

a. cyanosis

b. pallor

c. stasis dermatitis

d. phlegmasia

A 157

C. Stasis dermatitis.

Q 158

Which physical finding is seen with arterial insufficiency more frequently than with venous stasis?

a. red or blue skin

b. pallor

c. brown skin discoloration

d. induration

A 158

B. Pallor.

All of these findings may be seen with venous stasis. Pallor is more commonly seen with arterial insufficiency but may be seen with venous stasis due to arterial spasm in acute iliofemoral deep venous thrombosis.

Oliver MA: Clinical evaluation. In Talbot SR, Oliver MA: *Techniques of Venous Imaging*. Pasadena, Davies Publishing, 1992, pp 27–36.

Q 159

A condition characterized by severe swelling of the leg secondary to acute iliofemoral deep venous thrombosis, without redness or cyanosis, is:

a. pitting edema

b. lipedema

c. phlegmasia alba dolens

d. cellulitis

A 159

C. Phlegmasia alba dolens.

This serious condition is caused by arterial spasms secondary to the extensive, acute deep iliofemoral venous thrombosis. Swelling and pain accompany the pallor.

▶ Rumwell C, McPharlin M: *Vascular Technology: An Illustrated Review*, 5th edition. Pasadena, Davies Publishing, 2015, p 290.

Q 160

A 59-year-old female presents with gradual onset of edema beginning at the dorsum of the foot and proceeding proximally. Leg elevation does not relieve the swelling. Which condition best explains her symptoms?

a. lymphedema

b. embolization

c. superficial venous thrombosis

d. arterial ischemia

A 160

A. Lymphedema.

Lymphedema may be congenital or acquired. Acquired lymphedema usually involves the entire lower extremity and may be associated with a minor event such as an insect bite, ankle sprain, or cutaneous infection. The edema is usually not associated with other symptoms. It begins at the dorsum of the foot and proceeds proximally. There is no cutaneous pigmentation, dermatitis, or ulceration as in venous edema, although long-term cases may show hyperkeratosis of the skin. Lymphedema can be further differentiated from venous edema because venous edema will improve quickly with leg elevation but lymphedema will not.

- Dixon MB, Bergan JJ: Lymphedema. In Fahey VA (ed): *Vascular Nursing*. Philadelphia, Saunders, 1988, pp 33–47.
- Strandness DE, Zierler RE: Exercise ankle pressure measurements in arterial disease. In Bernstein EF (ed): *Noninvasive Diagnostic Techniques in Vascular Disease*, 3rd edition. St. Louis, Mosby, 1985, pp 575–583.
- Felty CL, Rooke TW: Lymphedema. In Fahey VA (ed): *Vascular Nursing*, 4th edition. St. Louis, Saunders, 2004.

Q 161

How should the patient be positioned to facilitate visualization of varicose veins?

a. supine

b. prone

c. Trendelenburg

d. standing

A 161

D. Standing.

Q 162

Limitations of CW Doppler evaluation for deep venous thrombosis include all of the following **EXCEPT**:

a. Partial thrombus may not be detected.

b. Venous incompetence cannot be detected.

c. Well-collateralized thrombosis may show normal flow patterns.

d. Inaccurate results may be obtained with a bifid venous system.

A 162

B. This statement–"venous incompetence cannot be detected"–is **NOT** true. CW Doppler can be used to evaluate for venous incompetence.

▶ Rumwell C, McPharlin M: *Vascular Technology: An Illustrated Review*, 5th edition. Pasadena, Davies Publishing, 2015, pp 301–302.

Q 163

In the lower extremity, maximum flow return in the venous system is present with:

a. expiration
b. Valsalva maneuver
c. release of distal compression
d. inspiration

A 163

A. Expiration.

In the lower extremity, flow in the venous system is diminished or absent during inspiration and maximal during expiration. Flow may be increased by release of proximal compression or by distal augmentation.

Q 164

A pulsatile venous signal is associated with:

a. varicose veins
b. deep venous thrombosis
c. congestive heart failure
d. pulmonary embolism

A 164

C. Congestive heart failure.

▶ Rumwell C, McPharlin M: *Vascular Technology: An Illustrated Review*, 5th edition. Pasadena, Davies Publishing, 2015, p 306.

Q 165

Detection of venous flow reversal with compression proximal to the probe (closer to the heart) indicates:

a. venous thrombosis between the compression and site of Doppler interrogation

b. absence of venous thrombosis above the level of compression

c. valvular incompetence with reflux between the augmentation and the Doppler interrogation

d. functional valves between the augmentation and the Doppler interrogation

A 165

C. Valvular incompetence with reflux between the augmentation and the Doppler interrogation.

If augmentation of the Doppler signal occurs with proximal limb compression, then blood flow is being forced backward through the vein under examination. If there is a valve between the two points, valvular incompetence and reflux are indicated.

▸ Rumwell C, McPharlin M: *Vascular Technology: An Illustrated Review*, 5th edition. Pasadena, Davies Publishing, 2015, p 305.

Q 166

A continuous venous signal obtained with CW Doppler is commonly seen with:

a. normality
b. collateral flow
c. congestive heart failure
d. fluid overload

A 166

B. Collateral flow.

Q 167

During a Valsalva maneuver, the normal Doppler response for the femoral vein is:

a. augmentation

b. cessation of flow

c. no change in flow

d. increased pulsatility of the venous signal

A 167

B. Cessation of flow.

A Valsalva maneuver is performed by the patient taking in a breath and then bearing down as if to have a bowel movement. This maneuver can be performed to evaluate for valvular competency. Normally, flow ceases during a Valsalva maneuver. If flow persists or increases, the valves between the groin and the area of interrogation are incompetent.

- Rumwell C, McPharlin M: *Vascular Technology: An Illustrated Review*, 5th edition. Pasadena, Davies Publishing, 2015, p 280.

Q 168

With calf compression, augmentation of the Doppler signal in the femoral vein indicates:

a. incompetent valves

b. reflux

c. normality

d. deep venous thrombosis in the popliteal vein

A 168

C. Normality.

Q 169

How should the patient be positioned for duplex evaluation of the lower extremity veins?

a. Trendelenburg

b. standing

c. decubitus

d. reverse Trendelenburg

A 169

D. Reverse Trendelenburg.

In a reverse Trendelenburg position, the bed is tilted 10°–20° with the feet lower than the head. This position promotes pooling of the blood within the veins, enlarging them and making them easier to visualize.

▶ Rumwell C, McPharlin M: *Vascular Technology: An Illustrated Review*, 5th edition. Pasadena, Davies Publishing, 2015, p 310.

Q 170

What vessels are seen with duplex ultrasound at the level of the inguinal ligament?

a. external iliac vein, internal iliac vein

b. femoral vein, superficial femoral artery, deep femoral artery

c. external iliac vein, internal iliac artery

d. common femoral vein, common femoral artery

A 170

D. Common femoral vein, common femoral artery.

Q 171

The saphenofemoral junction is identified by duplex sonography:

a. at the level of the knee
b. at the mid thigh
c. in the adductor canal
d. near the inguinal ligament

A 171

D. Near the inguinal ligament.

Q 172

If the great saphenous vein is **NOT** identified at the appropriate location, the examiner should:

a. use a posterior approach

b. decrease probe pressure

c. use a lateral approach

d. increase probe pressure

DAVIES
Registry Reviews & Study Aids

A 172

B. Decrease probe pressure.

Too much probe pressure is the mistake most commonly responsible for a failure to visualize the great saphenous or other superficial veins. These vessels are easily compressed by the weight of the probe resting on the skin.

- Talbot SR: Venous imaging technique. In Talbot SR, Oliver MA: *Techniques of Venous Imaging*. Pasadena, Davies Publishing, 1992, pp 59–118.

Q 173

Which veins located within the calf muscle are a common site of thrombus formation?

a. geniculate veins

b. femoral canal perforators (Hunter's veins)

c. soleal veins

d. anterior tibial veins

A 173

C. Soleal veins.

The soleal veins are located in the calf within the soleal muscle. They are a common site of thrombus formation. The soleal veins do not communicate with the superficial venous system; they empty into either the peroneal veins or the posterior tibial veins.

▸ Talbot SR: Venous imaging technique. In Talbot SR, Oliver MA: *Techniques of Venous Imaging*. Pasadena, Davies Publishing, 1992, pp 59–118.

Q 174

The main purpose of probe compression in duplex sonography is to:

a. rule out the presence of thrombus
b. differentiate between superficial and deep veins
c. rule out incompetent valves
d. differentiate between veins and arteries

A 174

A. Rule out the presence of thrombus.

Q 175

This image shows a thrombosed vein adjacent to the common carotid artery. What vein is being imaged?

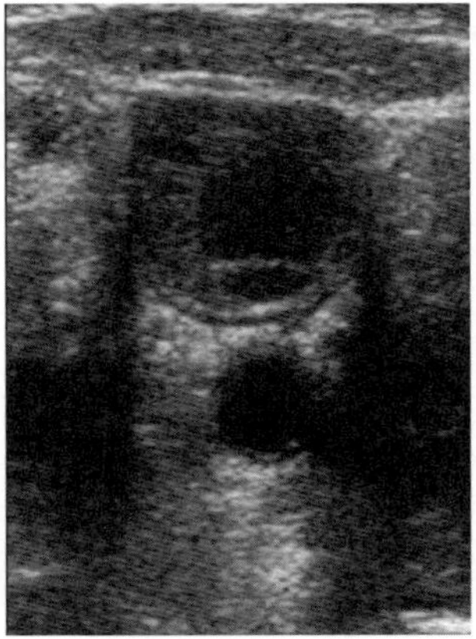

a. subclavian vein

b. internal jugular vein

c. innominate vein

d. external jugular vein

DAVIES Registry Reviews & Study Aids

A 175

B. Internal jugular vein.

The internal jugular vein courses with the common carotid artery. The external jugular vein does not accompany an artery.

▸ Talbot SR: Venous imaging technique. In Talbot SR, Oliver MA: *Techniques of Venous Imaging*. Pasadena, Davies Publishing, 1992, pp 59–118.

Q 176

Which color Doppler pattern is seen with valvular incompetency?

a. A reversal of color is seen with distal compression.
b. Color Doppler cannot detect valvular incompetency.
c. There is no change in color with proximal compression.
d. A reversal of color is seen with the Valsalva maneuver.

DAVIES Registry Reviews & Study Aids

A 176

D. A reversal of color is seen with the Valsalva maneuver.

Both proximal compression and the Valsalva maneuver can be used to rule out valvular incompetency. If a reversal of color is seen (from red to blue or blue to red) with either proximal compression or a Valsalva maneuver, valvular incompetency is suspected.

▶ Talbot SR: Venous imaging technique. In Talbot SR, Oliver MA: *Techniques of Venous Imaging*. Pasadena, Davies Publishing, 1992, pp 59–118.

Q 177

A technologist performing a venous study on the lower extremity notes that color Doppler does **NOT** demonstrate the calf veins filling spontaneously. What technical factors could be adjusted to improve color saturation?

a. increase color filter, decrease color pulse repetition frequency, increase color gain

b. increase color filter, increase color pulse repetition frequency, increase color gain

c. decrease color filter, increase color pulse repetition frequency, decrease color gain

d. decrease color filter, decrease color pulse repetition frequency, increase color gain

A 177

D. Decrease color filter, decrease color pulse repetition frequency (PRF), increase color gain.

The flow in the calf veins is very slow and may not be detected at default color settings. To sensitize the color system to detect slow-moving blood flow, both the color PRF and the wall filter should be decreased. Increasing the color gain will amplify the signal that is received and increase the display of color.

Q 178

In venous ultrasound, how is probe compression best performed?

a. in B-mode in a transverse orientation
b. in color mode in a transverse orientation
c. in B-mode in a sagittal orientation
d. in color mode in a sagittal orientation

A 178

A. In B-mode in a transverse orientation.

- Oliver MA: Doppler color flow imaging. In Talbot SR, Oliver MA: *Techniques of Venous Imaging*. Pasadena, Davies Publishing, 1992, pp 119–134.
- Rumwell C, McPharlin M: *Vascular Technology: An Illustrated Review*, 5th edition. Pasadena, Davies Publishing, 2015, pp 310–312.
- Ridgway DP: *Introduction to Vascular Scanning: A Guide for the Complete Beginner*, 4th edition. Pasadena, Davies Publishing, 2014, pp 205–212.

Q 179

Which characteristics below are associated with acute thrombus?

a. poorly attached, dilated vein, brightly echogenic, irregular borders
b. large collateral veins, contracted vein, brightly echogenic, irregular borders
c. poorly attached, dilated vein, hypoechoic, smooth borders
d. contracted vein, large collateral veins, hypoechoic, poorly attached

A 179

C. Poorly attached, dilated vein, hypoechoic, smooth borders.

These are all characteristics of acute thrombosis as opposed to chronic thrombosis. Other characteristics of acute thrombosis include a spongy texture and an incompressible vein.

- Talbot SR: Thrombus identification and characteristics. In Talbot SR, Oliver MA: *Techniques of Venous Imaging*. Pasadena, Davies Publishing, 1992, pp 37–58.

Q 180

Which characteristics below are associated with chronic thrombus?

a. poorly attached, dilated vein, hypoechoic, smooth borders

b. poorly attached, dilated vein, brightly echogenic, irregular borders

c. large collateral veins, contracted vein, brightly echogenic, irregular borders

d. contracted vein, large collateral veins, hypoechoic, poorly attached

A 180

C. Large collateral veins, contracted vein, brightly echogenic, irregular borders.

▸ Talbot SR: Thrombus identification and characteristics. In Talbot SR, Oliver MA: *Techniques of Venous Imaging*. Pasadena, Davies Publishing, 1992, pp 37–58.

Q 181

Coaptation of the supraclavicular subclavian vein is best performed by:

a. patient taking in a quick, deep breath
b. probe compression
c. Valsalva maneuver
d. distal limb compression

A 181

A. Patient taking in a quick, deep breath.

Because the subclavian vein is usually inaccessible to probe compression, coaptation can be performed by having the patient take in a quick, deep breath (sniff). If the walls are seen to coapt completely, that portion of the vein is judged to be thrombus-free.

▸ Talbot SR: Venous imaging technique. In Talbot SR, Oliver MA: *Techniques of Venous Imaging*. Pasadena, Davies Publishing, 1992, pp 59–118.

Q 182

A patient referred to the vascular lab presents with bilateral lower extremity edema and nephrotic syndrome. Within what vessel do you suspect thrombus?

a. inferior vena cava

b. left iliac vein

c. portal vein

d. splenic vein

DAVIES
Registry Reviews & Study Aids

A 182

A. Inferior vena cava.

IVC thrombus may produce bilateral leg swelling and recurrent pulmonary embolus. Nephrotic syndrome may occur if the thrombus is located at the level of the renal veins.

Q 183

Which is an advantage of color Doppler imaging over B-mode imaging alone in evaluation of the venous system?

a. Recanalized thrombi are more readily apparent.

b. Partially occluding thrombi are better detected.

c. Venous collaterals are more readily visualized.

d. All of the above.

A 183

D. All of the above.

Q 184

What is the normal Doppler response for the femoral vein immediately following a Valsalva maneuver?

a. augmentation

b. increased pulsatility of the venous signal

c. no change in flow

d. cessation of flow

A 184

A. Augmentation.

Immediately following a Valsalva maneuver, the venous flow will be augmented because blood can now course proximal.

▶ Rumwell C, McPharlin M: *Vascular Technology: An Illustrated Review*, 5th edition. Pasadena, Davies Publishing, 2015, p 305.

Q 185

A 48-year-old male is referred to the vascular lab to rule out the presence of a Baker's cyst. What anatomy would be imaged in this study?

a. Morison's pouch
b. Hunter's canal
c. popliteal fossa
d. subclavicular area

A 185

C. Popliteal fossa.

A Baker's cyst is seen as an anechoic area or area of mixed echogenicity in the popliteal fossa. It is separate from the artery and vein and does not fill with color Doppler. Also known as popliteal cysts, Baker's cysts are collections of synovial fluid in a sac posterior to the knee, although they may dissect down into the calf area. They can be quite painful.

▶ Talbot SR: Thrombus identification and characteristics. In Talbot SR, Oliver MA: *Techniques of Venous Imaging*. Pasadena, Davies Publishing, 1992, pp 37–58.

Q 186

Which vessels would be the most difficult to coapt with probe compression in cross section?

a. confluence of the femoral and saphenous vein
b. posterior tibial vein above the medial malleolus
c. femoral vein at the adductor canal
d. peroneal veins in the mid calf

A 186

C. Femoral vein at the adductor canal.

The femoral vein is sometimes difficult to visualize and/or compress at the level of the adductor canal. Compression can be made easier by the simple technique of placing one hand behind the leg and pressing upward while also pushing down with the other hand on the probe. Color Doppler can also be useful here to confirm patency of the vein.

▶ Ridgway DP: *Introduction to Vascular Scanning: A Guide for the Complete Beginner*, 4th edition. Pasadena, Davies Publishing, 2014, p 212.

Q 187

On a duplex examination of a 45-year-old male, a thrombus is seen in one of the gastrocnemius veins. Which vein would most likely be involved in the propagation of this thrombus?

a. common femoral

b. popliteal

c. soleal

d. anterior tibial

A 187

B. Popliteal.

The gastrocnemius veins are located around the knee and drain into the popliteal vein.

Q 188

What is the effect of expiration on a Doppler waveform obtained in the axillary vein?

a. augmentation

b. no effect

c. cessation

d. reversal

A 188

C. Cessation.

During expiration, venous flow from the lower extremities increases, whereas venous flow in the upper extremities stops.

▶ Rumwell C, McPharlin M: *Vascular Technology: An Illustrated Review*, 5th edition. Pasadena, Davies Publishing, 2015, p 280.

Q 189

A venous refill time that is less than 20 seconds without a tourniquet and less than 20 seconds with a tourniquet applied below the knee is consistent with:

a. normality
b. insufficiency of the deep and superficial systems
c. reflux in the great saphenous vein
d. reflux in the small saphenous vein

A 189

B. Insufficiency of the deep and superficial systems.

A normal venous refill time (VRT) measures ≥20 seconds. A VRT of <20 seconds without the tourniquet in conjunction with a VRT of >20 seconds with a tourniquet below the knee is consistent with reflux in the small saphenous vein. A VRT of <20 seconds without the tourniquet in conjunction with a VRT of >20 seconds with a tourniquet above the knee is consistent with reflux in the great saphenous vein.

▶ Rumwell C, McPharlin M: *Vascular Technology: An Illustrated Review*, 5th edition. Pasadena, Davies Publishing, 2015, pp 294–296.

Q 190

This Doppler waveform was obtained in the femoral vein. The arrow is pointing to an augmented portion of the spectrum. This could be caused by:

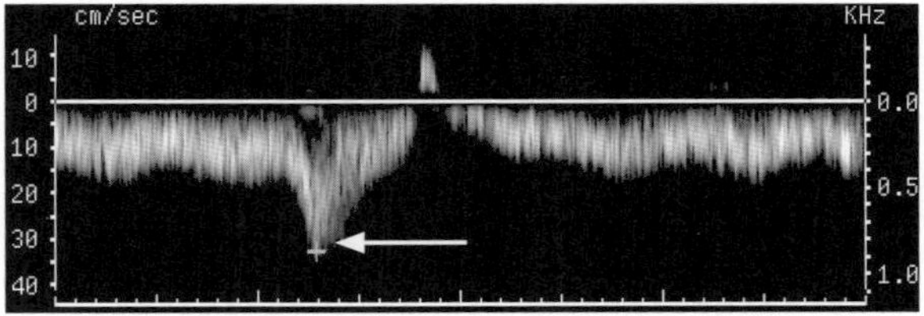

a. release of distal limb compression

b. proximal limb compression

c. distal limb compression

d. Valsalva maneuver

DAVIES
Registry Reviews & Study Aids

A 190

C. Distal limb compression.

With distal limb compression, blood is forced rapidly upstream past the point of Doppler sampling, thereby augmenting flow. This would not occur with release of the distal limb compression. Flow would cease with proximal limb compression or Valsalva maneuver.

▸ Rumwell C, McPharlin M: *Vascular Technology: An Illustrated Review*, 5th edition. Pasadena, Davies Publishing, 2015, p 305.

Q 191

Based on this image obtained in the internal jugular vein of a 34-year-old female, what diagnosis is most likely?

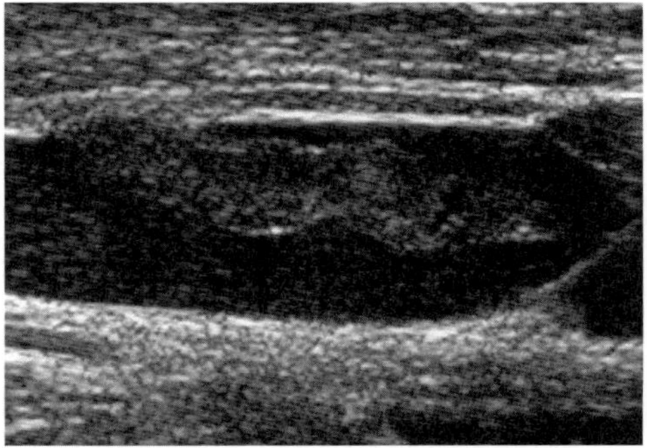

a. chronic thrombus

b. acute thrombus

c. valvular incompetence

d. rouleau formation without thrombus

A 191

B. Acute thrombus.

Q 192

The arrows in this image point to:

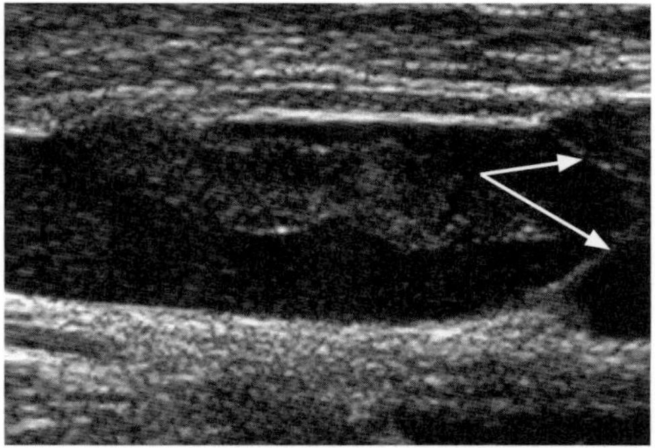

a. rouleau formation

b. valve leaflets

c. recanalized channels through thrombus

d. reverberation artifacts

DAVIES Registry Reviews & Study Aids

A 192

B. Valve leaflets.

Q 193

In ascending contrast venography of the lower extremity for diagnosis of DVT, the radiopaque material is typically injected into veins in the:

a. calf

b. arm

c. inguinal region

d. foot

A 193

D. Foot.

Q 194

In contrast venography, which finding would indicate the presence of a thrombus?

a. contrast extravasation

b. increase in opacity

c. filling defect

d. none of the above

A 194

C. Filling defect.

Q 195

Contrast venography is **NOT** frequently performed today because:

a. It is inaccurate.

b. There is a very high rate of severe allergic reactions.

c. Contrast venography cannot detect partially occlusive thrombus.

d. Duplex scanning is an accurate, noninvasive alternative.

A 195

D. Duplex scanning is an accurate, noninvasive alternative.

The limitations of contrast venography include the risk of severe allergic reactions, relatively high expense, and patient discomfort.

▸ Rumwell C, McPharlin M: *Vascular Technology: An Illustrated Review*, 5th edition. Pasadena, Davies Publishing, 2015, pp 333–334.

Q 196

A nuclear medicine screening test that detects perfusion defects of the lungs is known as:

a. bird's nest filter

b. V/Q (ventilation quotient, aka ventilation perfusion) scan

c. Greenfield filter

d. ascending contrast venography

DAVIES
Registry Reviews & Study Aids

A 196

B. V/Q (ventilation quotient) scan.

Q 197

Your patient is scheduled for a venous ablation procedure to correct reflux of the great saphenous vein (GSV). To properly position the laser sheath or radiofrequency catheter for that procedure, you will use this important landmark:

a. superficial epigastric

b. superior external pudendal

c. anterior accessory

d. posterior accessory

A 197

A. Superficial epigastric.

- Rumwell C, McPharlin M: *Vascular Technology: An Illustrated Review*, 5th edition. Pasadena, Davies Publishing, 2015, p 345.

Q 198

You are providing ultrasound guidance for administration of tumescent anesthesia during a venous ablation procedure. What is the preferred size of the zone of local anesthesia around the vein to be treated, e.g., the great saphenous vein?

a. 5 mm

b. 10 mm

c. 15 mm

d. 20 mm

A 198

B. 10 mm.

- Rumwell C, McPharlin M: *Vascular Technology: An Illustrated Review*, 5th edition. Pasadena, Davies Publishing, 2015, p 346.

Q 199

Following radiofrequency or laser ablation of the great saphenous vein (GSV), propagation of thrombus may be evident in the deep venous system. Which of the following statements about that event is most accurate?

a. It is an expected finding that does not need to be treated.

b. It may be described as endovenous heat-induced thrombus.

c. Propagation of the thrombus into the deep system requires ligation of the GSV.

d. Extension of thrombus into the deep system suggests a failure to successfully ablate the GSV.

A 199

C. Propagation of the thrombus into the deep system requires ligation of the GSV.

▶ Rumwell C, McPharlin M: *Vascular Technology: An Illustrated Review*, 5th edition. Pasadena, Davies Publishing, 2015, p 351.

Q 200

Your patient presents with chronic ankle and calf edema and undergoes a PPG test that suggests significant valvular incompetence. When the test is repeated, a tourniquet is applied around the leg just below the knee. There is no appreciable change in the tracing. What does this finding suggest?

a. superficial valvular incompetence only

b. deep venous valvular incompetence

c. equivocal results

d. nonvenous causes of the edema

A 200

B. Deep venous valvular incompetence.

The tourniquet eliminates the influence of the superficial system. Had the tracing reverted to normal with the tourniquet, the superficial system would then be implicated. In this case it is the deep veins–instead of or in addition to the superficial veins–that appear to be incompetent.

▶ Rumwell CB, McPharlin M: *Vascular Technology: An Illustrated Review*, 5th edition. Pasadena, Davies Publishing, 2015, p 296.

Q 201

You are performing photoplethysmography on a patient with chronic ankle and calf edema. The PPG sensor is placed slightly proximal to the medial malleolus, and the patient dorsiflexes five times, then relaxes, resulting in this tracing. What does it suggest?

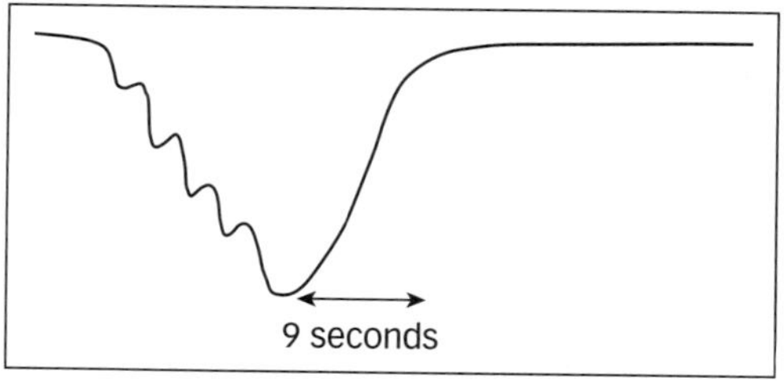

a. within normal limits
b. not venous but arterial insufficiency
c. significant valvular incompetence
d. acute deep vein thrombosis

A 201

C. Significant valvular incompetence.

The PPG tracing is a reflection of intravenous pressure. The dorsiflexions reduce intravenous pressure to a minimum, and the return to original pressure should result only from inflow from capillaries and therefore take at least 20 seconds. A rapid return like this one suggests that blood is refluxing because of valvular incompetence.

- Rumwell CB, McPharlin M: *Vascular Technology: An Illustrated Review*, 5th edition. Pasadena, Davies Publishing, 2015, p 296.

Q 202

Photoplethysmography was performed on your patient. Venous refilling time was 10 seconds without a tourniquet applied and 25 seconds with a tourniquet applied to the lower thigh. What is the diagnosis?

a. deep valvular insufficiency
b. superficial venous thrombosis
c. deep venous thrombosis
d. superficial valvular insufficiency

A 202

D. Superficial valvular insufficiency.

The tourniquet took the superficial system out of the picture, which returned the result to normal. Therefore, the superficial system caused the rapid refill.

▶ Rumwell CB, McPharlin M: *Vascular Technology: An Illustrated Review*, 5th edition. Pasadena, Davies Publishing, 2015, p 296.

Q 203

Which of the following is a cause of blue toe syndrome?

a. venous thrombosis of the pedal veins
b. hyperemic flow from arteriovenous fistulas
c. congenital absence of the dorsalis pedis artery
d. embolization from proximal arteries

A 203

D. Embolization from proximal arteries.

▶ Rumwell C, McPharlin M: *Vascular Technology: An Illustrated Review*, 5th edition. Pasadena, Davies Publishing, 2015, p 48.

Q 204

In which syndrome does recurrent digital vasospasm occur in response to cold exposure or emotional stress?

a. Buerger's syndrome

b. Raynaud's syndrome

c. Takayasu's syndrome

d. thoracic outlet syndrome

A 204

B. Raynaud's syndrome.

Also known as *Raynaud's phenomenon*, this vasospastic disorder most commonly occurs in women following exposure to cold or emotional stress. Classically, Raynaud's syndrome is characterized by profound skin pallor and numbness. Cyanosis occurs with warming of the digits, and then erythema follows accompanied by a burning pain.

▸ Rumwell C, McPharlin M: *Vascular Technology: An Illustrated Review*, 5th edition. Pasadena, Davies Publishing, 2015, pp 46, 52–53, 111, 113.

Q 205

Which disease involves thrombosis of the small or medium-sized arteries of the extremities and occurs predominantly in male smokers?

a. Allen's disease

b. Buerger's disease

c. Raynaud's disease

d. thoracic outlet disease

A 205

B. Buerger's disease.

Buerger's disease is the most common of the several types of arteritis (inflammation of the arterial wall). Other types include Takayasu's arteritis, temporal arteritis, and polyarteritis. Buerger's disease is also known as *thromboangiitis obliterans.* It occurs mainly in men younger than 40 years of age and is strongly associated with heavy cigarette smoking. Patients experience rest pain and ischemic ulceration early in the disease and present with occlusions of the distal-most arteries (e.g., fingers and toes). The presentation can be dramatic, often including both ulceration and gangrene.

▶ Rumwell C, McPharlin M: *Vascular Technology: An Illustrated Review*, 5th edition. Pasadena, Davies Publishing, 2015, pp 50–51.

Q 206

Which of these conditions most commonly affects the subclavian, renal, and carotid arteries and the ascending aorta and predominantly affects females?

a. Takayasu's arteritis

b. temporal arteritis

c. polyarteritis nodosa

d. Kawasaki disease

A 206

A. Takayasu's arteritis.

Takayasu's arteritis is a chronic inflammatory process that primarily affects the aorta and its major branches. The carotid bulb and proximal internal carotid artery are usually spared. More than 95% of affected patients are females in the second or third decade of life. Stenoses in these patients tend to be long, tapered, and smooth. These patients often have hypertension due to involvement of the renal arteries. Stroke is the presenting symptom in 14% of patients. Ultrasound findings include homogeneous segmental wall thickening, which has been termed the "macaroni" sign when viewed in transverse. This is usually associated with increased flow velocity through the affected area. In cerebrovascular involvement, homogeneous segmental wall thickening is usually limited to the common carotid and subclavian arteries. It is not uncommon to find occlusion of the common carotid artery with reversed flow from the ipsilateral external carotid artery to the patent ipsilateral internal carotid.

- Rumwell C, McPharlin M: *Vascular Technology: An Illustrated Review*, 5th edition. Pasadena, Davies Publishing, 2015, pp 251–252.
- Sun Y, Yip PK, Jeng JS, et al: Ultrasonographic study and long-term follow-up of Takayasu's arteritis. Stroke 27:2178–2182, 1996.

Q 207

Hemorrhage within the layers of the arterial wall is known as:

a. ulceration
b. pseudoaneurysm
c. arteriovenous fistula
d. dissection

A 207

D. Dissection.

Dissection refers to hemorrhage within the wall of an artery. The hemorrhage may be localized within the media, may be located between the intima and media, or may involve the adventitia. When extravasated blood elevates the intima, an intimal flap results. Two lumina (a true and a false channel) can result, separated by the intimal flap. Usually there are multiple connections between the true and false lumina. Thrombosis of one lumen can occur, narrowing the artery. Dissections can occur spontaneously or as the result of trauma. Trauma may be either blunt or penetrating. Spontaneous dissections are related to systemic hypertension, fibromuscular dysplasia, cystic medial necrosis, Marfan syndrome, or type IV Ehlers-Danlos syndrome. Sonographic findings include visualization of a mobile intimal flap or a long, smooth, and tapering stenosis suggesting thrombosis. Color Doppler can be useful in delineating flow within two distinct channels in the artery or demonstrating absence of flow in one lumen.

▸ Provenzale JM: Dissection of the internal carotid and vertebral arteries: imaging features. AJR 165:1099–1104, 1995.

Q 208

What is the name of the nonatherosclerotic, noninflammatory, occlusive, and aneurysmal disorder that primarily affects women and is referred to as a "string of beads" or "string of pearls"?

a. Takayasu's disease

b. fibromuscular dysplasia

c. polyarteritis nodosa

d. mycotic aneurysm

DAVIES
Registry Reviews & Study Aids

A 208

B. Fibromuscular dysplasia.

Approximately 90% of cases of fibromuscular dysplasia occur in women. It most frequently affects the renal arteries, with carotid artery involvement being the next most common. Renal involvement may result in renovascular hypertension. Carotid involvement is most often benign, and most patients remain asymptomatic. Fewer than 10% of carotid lesions produce symptoms. One-half of patients with carotid involvement will have the disease in both carotid arteries. From 25% to 50% of patients with carotid fibromuscular dysplasia will have associated renal artery fibromuscular dysplasia. The vertebral artery is less frequently involved.

- Rumwell C, McPharlin M: *Vascular Technology: An Illustrated Review*, 5th edition. Pasadena, Davies Publishing, 2015, pp 142, 177, 215–216, 233, 255.
- Hurlbert SN, Krupski WC: Carotid artery disease in women. Semin Vasc Surg 8:268–276, 1995.

Q 209

Which syndrome below is caused by swelling within the osteofascial compartments of the leg or arm and results in decreased vascular perfusion?

a. thoracic outlet syndrome

b. Raynaud's syndrome

c. compartment syndrome

d. Marfan syndrome

A 209

C. Compartment syndrome.

This condition most commonly occurs after revascularization following prolonged ischemia, but may also develop secondary to external compression or bleeding within the compartment.

▶ Rumwell C, McPharlin M: *Vascular Technology: An Illustrated Review*, 5th edition. Pasadena, Davies Publishing, 2015, pp 167–168.

Q 210

Which syndrome results in medial displacement of the vessel due to compression by fibrous bands or the medial head of the gastrocnemius muscle?

a. thoracic outlet syndrome

b. compartment syndrome

c. adductor canal compression syndrome

d. popliteal entrapment syndrome

A 210

D. Popliteal entrapment syndrome.

This syndrome occurs when the artery is compressed by the medial head of the gastrocnemius muscle or fibrous bands. The popliteal artery is usually dislocated medially. Popliteal entrapment syndrome is more common in young men and occurs bilaterally in up to one-third of cases. The trauma caused to the artery can result in the development of aneurysm, thrombosis, atherosclerosis, or embolic phenomena. Symptoms include intermittent claudication. Doppler findings include diminished or altered waveforms with knee extension, active plantar flexion, or passive dorsiflexion of the foot.

▸ Rumwell C, McPharlin M: *Vascular Technology: An Illustrated Review*, 5th edition. Pasadena, Davies Publishing, 2015, pp 53, 169–170.

Q 211

Which of the following may be a source of emboli?

a. ulcerated atherosclerotic plaque

b. mural thrombus within an aneurysm

c. cardiac dysrhythmias

d. all of the above

DAVIES
Registry Reviews & Study Aids

A 211

D. All of the above.

An embolus is a plug—a foreign object—carried along in the bloodstream. It may be solid, liquid, or gaseous and may arise within the body or be introduced from without. Most commonly, an embolus is a fragment of thrombus or plaque that has dislodged from its origin and coursed distally in the bloodstream before obstructing a small vessel. It may arise from ulcerative atherosclerotic plaque, mural thrombus in an aneurysm, or the heart.

Q 212

Which of the following is **NOT** a risk factor for development of atherosclerotic disease?

a. diabetes mellitus

b. male sex

c. underweight

d. hypertension

A 212

C. Underweight.

Dominant risk factors for the development of atherosclerotic disease include increasing age, male sex, cigarette smoking, diabetes mellitus, obesity, hyperlipidemia, hypertension, and positive family history of atherosclerotic disease.

- Rumwell C, McPharlin M: *Vascular Technology: An Illustrated Review*, 5th edition. Pasadena, Davies Publishing, 2015, pp 53, 45–51.
- Parker BC, Bandyk DF, Mills JL, et al: Clinical evaluation of occlusive peripheral vascular disease. In Strandness DE, van Breda A (eds): *Vascular Diseases: Surgical and Interventional Therapy*. New York, Churchill Livingstone, 1994, pp 423–431.

Q 213

What is the most serious risk from femoropopliteal aneurysms?

a. fistula

b. rupture

c. embolization

d. infection

A 213

C. Embolization.

The most serious risk from femoropopliteal aneurysms is lower limb ischemia from thrombosis or embolization. The most important features of these aneurysms are thrombus content and vessel tortuosity. These factors may result in sudden thrombosis and severe ischemia of the lower limb. The most serious risk of aortic aneurysms is rupture.

▸ Ballard DJ, Hallett JW: Natural history of aneurysms. In Strandness DE, van Breda A (eds): *Vascular Diseases: Surgical and Interventional Therapy*. New York, Churchill Livingstone, 1994, pp 565–569.

Q 214

Which of these statements about primary Raynaud's phenomenon is correct?

a. It results from ischemia caused by distal arterial spasm.
b. It relates to vasodilation of a healthy vessel.
c. It can be the first manifestation of thromboangiitis obliterans.
d. It is often evident after an acute arterial occlusion.

DAVIES
Registry Reviews & Study Aids

A 214

A. It results from ischemia caused by distal arterial spasm.

▶ Rumwell C, McPharlin M: *Vascular Technology: An Illustrated Review*, 5th edition. Pasadena, Davies Publishing, 2015, p 52.

Q 215

What symptom involves cramping muscle pain that is induced by exercise and relieved by rest?

a. claudication

b. rest pain

c. bruit

d. thrill

A 215

A. Claudication.

▸ Rumwell C, McPharlin M: *Vascular Technology: An Illustrated Review*, 5th edition. Pasadena, Davies Publishing, 2015, pp 45–46.

Q 216

What severe symptom of decreased blood perfusion is aggravated by elevation, is relieved by dependency, and often occurs when the patient goes to bed at night?

a. claudication

b. cyanosis

c. postprandial pain

d. rest pain

DAVIES
Registry Reviews & Study Aids

A 216

D. Rest pain.

▶ Rumwell C, McPharlin M: *Vascular Technology: An Illustrated Review*, 5th edition. Pasadena, Davies Publishing, 2015, p 46.

Q 217

A smooth, painful ulcer located on the dorsum of the foot is most likely a(n):

a. ischemic ulcer
b. stasis ulcer
c. lymphedema ulcer
d. neurotrophic ulcer

A 217

A. Ischemic ulcer.

Ischemic ulcers are most commonly located over pressure points such as the toe, heel, or dorsum of the foot. They may occur spontaneously or with trauma. Pain is often severe at night and is relieved by placing the extremity in a dependent position. The ulcer base is usually pale and the edge is definitive. The skin around it is atrophic or inflamed. Other trophic changes seen with arterial insufficiency include loss of hair on the affected extremity, shiny and smooth skin, thick brittle nails, and tapering of the toes or fingers. *Stasis ulcers* are caused by venous stasis in chronic venous insufficiency. They tend to occur over the medial distal third of the leg (gaiter zone). Pain is mild and is relieved by elevating the affected extremity. The ulcer edge appears uneven and the skin around the ulcer may show a brownish discoloration caused by hemosiderin deposits from the breakdown of red blood cells. *Neurotrophic ulcers* are associated with diabetes. They occur spontaneously and are located on the sole of the foot under calluses or on pressure points. They do not cause pain. The ulcer edge is definitive and the skin around it is callous.

▸ Rumwell C, McPharlin M: *Vascular Technology: An Illustrated Review*, 5th edition. Pasadena, Davies Publishing, 2015, p 54.

Q 218

Which term describes a pale skin color due to insufficient blood flow?

a. cyanosis

b. rubella

c. rubor

d. pallor

A 218

D. Pallor.

▶ Rumwell C, McPharlin M: *Vascular Technology: An Illustrated Review*, 5th edition. Pasadena, Davies Publishing, 2015, p 54.

Q 219

Which of these statements about bruits is **NOT** true?

a. A bruit is a low-frequency sound heard on auscultation.

b. A prominent bruit will be heard over an arterial occlusion.

c. The absence of a bruit cannot rule out disease.

d. A bruit persisting through diastole is usually associated with severe stenosis.

DAVIES Registry Reviews & Study Aids

A 219

B. This statement–"a prominent bruit will be heard over an arterial occlusion"–is **NOT** true.

A bruit is a vibratory reaction in the tissue distal to a stenosis. It will not be present with complete occlusion or trickle flow in high-grade stenosis, but its absence does not rule out vascular disease, including severe stenosis.

▸ Rumwell C, McPharlin M: *Vascular Technology: An Illustrated Review*, 5th edition. Pasadena, Davies Publishing, 2015, p 56.

Q 220

A patient presents to the vascular lab with a history of recent brachial artery catheterization and a palpable thrill over the brachial artery. Which diagnosis is most likely?

a. complete thrombosis of the brachial artery

b. deep venous thrombosis of the brachial vein

c. hematoma surrounding the brachial artery

d. arteriovenous fistula involving the brachial artery and vein

A 220

D. Arteriovenous fistula involving the brachial artery and vein.

A vascular thrill is a palpable vibration over an artery. It indicates a high-flow state with turbulence and is commonly felt over a fistula site. In this case, the patient reports a recent brachial artery catheterization. Complications of arterial catheterization include arteriovenous fistula, pseudoaneurysm, hematoma, and thrombosis. Of these, only the fistula and possibly the pseudoaneurysm will produce a palpable thrill.

▶ Rumwell C, McPharlin M: *Vascular Technology: An Illustrated Review*, 5th edition. Pasadena, Davies Publishing, 2015, pp 56, 120, 165–167.

Q 221

The best way for a vascular technologist to palpate a pulse is to:

a. place the back of his hand over the pulse site
b. place his thumb over the pulse site
c. place his fingertips over the pulse site
d. push hard over the pulse site with both hands

DAVIES
Registry Reviews & Study Aids

A 221

C. Place his fingertips over the pulse site.

When the thumb is used to palpate a pulse, the examiner cannot determine if the origin of the pulse is from the patient or himself. The best way to palpate a pulse is to place your fingertips over the pulse site.

Q 222

A pulse palpated in the groove behind the medial malleolus of the ankle corresponds to which artery?

a. anterior tibial artery

b. peroneal artery

c. posterior tibial artery

d. plantar artery

DAVIES Registry Reviews & Study Aids

A 222

C. Posterior tibial artery.

Palpable pulses include the aorta and femoral, popliteal, dorsalis pedis, and posterior tibial arteries. The peroneal artery cannot be palpated.

▶ Fahey VA: Clinical assessment of the vascular system. In Fahey VA (ed): *Vascular Nursing*, 4th edition. St. Louis, Saunders, 2004, pp 49–71.

Q 223

What is indicated by the presence of a bruit?

a. arterial occlusion directly beneath the point of auscultation

b. the absence of arterial disease

c. arterial stenosis proximal to the point of auscultation

d. venous thrombosis

DAVIES
Registry Reviews & Study Aids

A 223

C. Arterial stenosis proximal to the point of auscultation.

See answer 219.

Q 224

A patient with a history of tibial artery surgical repair now presents with foot drop, muscle necrosis, and severe pain. What diagnosis is suspected?

a. compartment syndrome

b. pseudoaneurysm

c. Raynaud's syndrome

d. arteriovenous fistula

A 224

A. Compartment syndrome.

Q 225

Following repair of injuries to the anterior tibial artery after a motor vehicle accident, your patient complains of weakness in the calf muscle, paresthesia, and pain on passive stretching of the calf muscle. What condition does this suggest?

a. cystic adventitial disease

b. compartment syndrome

c. Paget-Schroetter syndrome

d. acute arterial occlusion

A 225

B. Compartment syndrome.

▸ Rumwell C, McPharlin M: *Vascular Technology: An Illustrated Review*, 5th edition. Pasadena, Davies Publishing, 2015, pp 167–168.

Q 226

Which one of the following is always **TRUE** of patients who suffer from intermittent claudication?

a. Peripheral blood flow is reduced at rest.
b. There is pressure drop distal to the obstructed segment after exercise.
c. Marked peripheral vasoconstriction occurs in response to exercise.
d. There is always a pressure drop distal to the obstructed segment at rest.

A 226

B. There is pressure drop distal to the obstructed segment after exercise.

Peripheral flow is generally maintained at rest by compensatory vasodilatation distally. Exercise causes pronounced vasodilatation, greatly increasing flow. Although claudicators usually have a reduced resting pressure, they can sometimes have equivocal or even essentially normal ABIs at rest. Thus some form of challenge (exercise or postocclusive reactive hyperemia) might be required to provoke a pressure drop.

- Rumwell C, McPharlin M: *Vascular Technology: An Illustrated Review*, 5th edition. Pasadena, Davies Publishing, 2015, p 170.
- Sumner DS: Essential hemodynamic principles. In Rutherford RB (ed): *Vascular Surgery*, 5th edition. Philadelphia, Saunders, 2000, p 84.

Q 227

In the presence of arterial obstructive disease and distal ischemia:

a. vasoconstriction increases, and distal resistance increases

b. vasodilatation increases, and distal resistance decreases

c. vasoconstriction increases, and distal resistance decreases

d. vasodilatation decreases, and distal resistance decreases

A 227

B. Vasodilatation increases, and distal resistance decreases.

The body attempts to increase nutritive blood flow to the extremity by vasodilatation and the subsequent decrease of peripheral resistance. The drop in distal pressure is a result of the increased segmental resistance and “stealing” of blood to the large muscle groups.

▸ Carter SA: Role of pressure measurements. In Bernstein EF (ed): *Vascular Diagnosis*, 4th edition. St. Louis, Mosby, 1993, p 486.

Q 228

The vein most commonly used in the lower extremity as a reversed vein bypass graft is the:

a. cephalic vein
b. femoral vein
c. small saphenous vein
d. great saphenous vein

A 228

D. Great saphenous vein.

The great saphenous vein (GSV) is the vein of choice for reversed vein grafts in the lower extremity. If the GSV is unavailable, the cephalic, brachial, or small saphenous vein may be used.

- Rumwell C, McPharlin M: *Vascular Technology: An Illustrated Review*, 5th edition. Pasadena, Davies Publishing, 2015, pp 131–132.
- Ridgway DP: *Introduction to Vascular Scanning: A Guide for the Complete Beginner*, 4th edition. Pasadena, Davies Publishing, 2014, pp 266–270.

Q 229

With which type of bypass graft will there be a size discrepancy between the graft and the native artery at both the proximal and distal anastomotic sites?

a. in situ vein graft
b. reversed vein graft
c. synthetic graft
d. Greenfield graft

A 229

B. Reversed vein graft.

In a reversed vein graft, the vein (usually the great saphenous vein) is surgically lifted from its bed and reversed before being attached to the normal portion of the native artery. An advantage of this technique is that the venous valves are oriented in the direction of blood flow. Additionally, all vein branches are easily ligated since the entire vein has been exposed during surgery. A disadvantage is the caliber discrepancy between the graft and the native artery at both anastomotic sites. This occurs because the saphenous vein is normally larger in the thigh and smaller at the ankle. Reversing the vein results in the smaller end being connected to the largest part of the native artery and the larger end being connected to the smallest part of the native artery.

- Rumwell C, McPharlin M: *Vascular Technology: An Illustrated Review*, 5th edition. Pasadena, Davies Publishing, 2015, pp 131–132.
- Polak JF: Arterial sonography: efficacy for the diagnosis of arterial disease of the lower extremity. AJR 161:235–243, 1993.

Q 230

Which bypass graft would most likely be seen in a patient with bilateral common iliac artery obstruction?

a. femoral to posterior tibial artery

b. aortobifemoral

c. femoral to femoral

d. femoral to popliteal

A 230

B. Aortobifemoral.

Q 231

What is the most common form of nonsurgical intervention for focal atherosclerotic disease in the lower extremity?

a. atherectomy

b. thrombectomy

c. angioplasty

d. endarterectomy

DAVIES Registry Reviews & Study Aids

A 231

C. Angioplasty.

Also known as *balloon angioplasty* and *percutaneous transluminal angioplasty* (PTA), angioplasty is performed by inserting a balloon-tipped catheter into an artery, positioning the tip of the catheter within the stenotic segment to be dilated, and slowly inflating the balloon, which pushes the plaque against the vessel wall and enlarges the vessel lumen to a normal or nearly normal diameter. Often this enlarged lumen is then held open with a tiny metal mesh cylinder called a *stent.*

▶ Rumwell C, McPharlin M: *Vascular Technology: An Illustrated Review*, 5th edition. Pasadena, Davies Publishing, 2015, pp 183–192.

Q 232

What complication that may follow femoral artery catheterization involves a characteristic to-and-fro Doppler waveform seen within a tract leading to a perivascular hematoma?

a. arteriovenous fistula

b. occlusion

c. pseudoaneurysm

d. mycotic aneurysm

A 232

C. Pseudoaneurysm.

Pseudoaneurysms occur when a puncture site fails to close and blood escapes into the surrounding tissue, forming a perivascular hematoma. Color and spectral Doppler can be used to confirm the vascular nature of the mass and to identify the tract or neck leading from the native vessel to the pseudoaneurysm. The Doppler waveform obtained within the pseudoaneurysm will be turbulent. The Doppler waveform obtained from the neck will show a classic to-and-fro flow pattern with high velocities.

- Rumwell C, McPharlin M: *Vascular Technology: An Illustrated Review*, 5th edition. Pasadena, Davies Publishing, 2015, pp 49–50, 193–196.
- Hertz SM, Brener BJ: Ultrasound-guided pseudoaneurysm compression: efficacy after coronary stenting and angioplasty. J Vasc Surg 26:913–918, 1997.

Q 233

Which of the following is a late complication of extremity bypass grafts?

a. intimal hyperplasia
b. pseudoaneurysm
c. arteriovenous fistula
d. hematoma

A 233

A. Intimal hyperplasia.

Hematomas and pseudoaneurysms associated with extremity bypass grafts are usually seen in the immediate postoperative period. Arteriovenous fistulas occur because of failure to ligate a vein branch and are typically discovered as an early complication following surgery. Arteriovenous fistulas also may spontaneously open or close with the changing hemodynamics of the graft. Intimal hyperplasia is a late complication of bypass grafts resulting from the accumulation of smooth-muscle cells and matrix forming a fibrous thickening in the graft. This can occur either focally or diffusely and lead to stenosis. It tends to occur at the anastomotic sites, venous valve sites, and clamp sites.

- Rumwell C, McPharlin M: *Vascular Technology: An Illustrated Review*, 5th edition. Pasadena, Davies Publishing, 2015, p 186.
- Hertz SM, Brener BJ: Ultrasound-guided pseudoaneurysm compression: efficacy after coronary stenting and angioplasty. J Vasc Surg 26:913–918, 1997.
- Polak JF: Arterial sonography: efficacy for the diagnosis of arterial disease of the lower extremity. AJR 161:235–243, 1993.

Q 234

A technique whereby atherosclerotic plaque is mechanically removed by cutting or pulverizing it and then extracted by suction or downstream embolization is termed:

a. thrombectomy

b. angioplasty

c. atherectomy

d. endarterectomy

A 234

C. Atherectomy.

▶ Rumwell C, McPharlin M: *Vascular Technology: An Illustrated Review*, 5th edition. Pasadena, Davies Publishing, 2015, pp 192–193.

Q 235

What quantitative index is calculated by dividing the peak-to-peak frequency difference by the mean frequency?

a. resistive index

b. volume index

c. pulsatility index

d. acceleration index

DAVIES
Registry Reviews & Study Aids

A 235

C. Pulsatility index.

The *pulsatility index* (PI) is calculated by dividing the peak-to-peak frequency by the mean (average) frequency as depicted in the following equation:

$$PI = \frac{\text{Peak-to-Peak Frequency}}{\text{Mean Frequency}}$$

▶ Rumwell C, McPharlin M: *Vascular Technology: An Illustrated Review*, 5th edition. Pasadena, Davies Publishing, 2015, p 67.

Q 236

The measurement that helps in differentiating between inflow and outflow disease by determining the time between the onset of systole and the initial systolic peak is the:

a. acceleration time

b. volume flow

c. A/B ratio

d. resistive index

DAVIES
Registry Reviews & Study Aids

A 236

A. Acceleration time.

Acceleration time represents the time period between the onset of systole and the point of maximum peak velocity.

▶ Rumwell C, McPharlin M: *Vascular Technology: An Illustrated Review*, 5th edition. Pasadena, Davies Publishing, 2015, pp 66–68, p 148.

Q 237

Which method of Doppler display exhibits a gray-scale trace representing the entire range of reflected frequency shifts from the location of the sample volume?

a. spectral analysis

b. analog waveform

c. power Doppler

d. color flow

DAVIES Registry Reviews & Study Aids

A 237

A. Spectral analysis.

Q 238

What does a high-pitched signal heard on audible Doppler analysis always indicate?

a. the presence of high-velocity flow

b. high frequency shifts

c. the presence of a stenosis

d. a vessel kink

A 238

B. High frequency shifts.

A high frequency shift produces a higher-pitched signal. The magnitude of the Doppler frequency shift is determined not only by the speed of the flow but also by the angle at which the Doppler beam intersects the flow (the Doppler "look" angle) and the Doppler frequency. Since the Doppler frequency is constant during a given Doppler sampling, the two factors that can be responsible for increased pitch (frequency) are high blood flow velocity and decreased angle of incidence. This fact is demonstrated by the Doppler equation: Frequency shift $= 2 \text{ f V} \cos \theta \div \text{c}$, where f = operating frequency of the Doppler transducer, V = velocity of blood flow, $\cos \theta$ = cosine of Doppler "look" angle, c = speed of ultrasound in soft tissue (i.e., 1540 m/sec).

▶ Rumwell C, McPharlin M: *Vascular Technology: An Illustrated Review*, 5th edition. Pasadena, Davies Publishing, 2015, pp 51–68, 128–129.

Q 239

What should the patient's position be when you are taking ankle pressures?

a. sitting
b. standing
c. supine
d. reverse Trendelenburg

A 239

C. Supine.

Ankle pressures should be obtained with the patient supine and in a resting state.

▶ Rumwell C, McPharlin M: *Vascular Technology: An Illustrated Review*, 5th edition. Pasadena, Davies Publishing, 2015, pp 70–71.

Q 240

The cuff for obtaining pressures in the fingers should be what size?

a. 0.5–1 cm

b. 3 cm

c. 5 cm

d. 2–2.5 cm

A 240

D. 2–2.5 cm.

▶ Rumwell C, McPharlin M: *Vascular Technology: An Illustrated Review*, 5th edition. Pasadena, Davies Publishing, 2015, p 108.

Q 241

Which of the following correctly describes an advantage of pulsed-wave (PW) Doppler over continuous-wave (CW) Doppler?

a. PW Doppler is more accurate in measuring high velocities.
b. PW Doppler does not exhibit aliasing.
c. Echoes can be received from a specific depth with PW Doppler.
d. PW Doppler is more accurate in measuring low velocities.

A 241

C. Echoes can be received from a specific depth with PW Doppler.

This is termed *range-gating*. Since the speed of sound in tissue is known (1540 m/sec), the round-trip time to a specific depth (sample volume location) is easily determined. The system sends a pulse and then waits the calculated time to receive echoes only from the desired depth. This is not possible with CW Doppler, in which echoes are continually received from all moving interfaces encountered in the path of the beam.

Q 242

What is suggested by an acceleration time of less than 133 msec obtained in the femoral artery?

a. proximal iliac artery stenosis

b. the absence of significant iliac artery disease

c. distal femoral artery occlusion

d. pseudoaneurysm of the femoral artery

A 242

B. The absence of significant iliac artery disease.

A rapid upstroke in systole results in a short acceleration time. This pattern is consistent with normal inflow. A delayed upstroke occurs with significant inflow disease (stenosis proximal to the site of sampling).

▶ Rumwell C, McPharlin M: *Vascular Technology: An Illustrated Review*, 5th edition. Pasadena, Davies Publishing, 2015, pp 67–68.

Q 243

A disease in which segmental pressure studies may show falsely elevated Doppler pressures due to arterial wall calcification is:

a. diabetes mellitus

b. Takayasu's arteritis

c. Raynaud's syndrome

d. Marfan syndrome

DAVIES
Registry Reviews & Study Aids

A 243

A. Diabetes mellitus.

The vessels of patients with diabetes may be incompressible because of arterial wall calcification, a condition that leads to falsely elevated pressures.

▸ Rumwell C, McPharlin M: *Vascular Technology: An Illustrated Review*, 5th edition. Pasadena, Davies Publishing, 2015, pp 69, 75, 77, 82.

Q 244

The ankle/brachial index is calculated by dividing the ankle pressure by:

a. the highest of the two brachial pressures
b. the left brachial pressure
c. the lowest of the two brachial pressures
d. the right brachial pressure

A 244

A. The highest of the two brachial pressures.

▶ Rumwell C, McPharlin M: *Vascular Technology: An Illustrated Review*, 5th edition. Pasadena, Davies Publishing, 2015, pp 74–75.

Q 245

Using the four-cuff technique for segmental pressures, what is the relationship of normal high-thigh pressures and brachial pressure?

a. High-thigh pressures are not compared to brachial pressure.

b. They are equal.

c. High-thigh pressures are at least 30 mmHg less than brachial pressure.

d. High-thigh pressures are at least 30 mmHg greater than brachial pressure.

A 245

D. High-thigh pressures are at least 30 mmHg greater than brachial pressure.

Using the four-cuff technique for segmental pressures, the high-thigh cuff is small in diameter compared to the limb. This results in an artifactually elevated pressure at the high-thigh site. Therefore, normal pressures obtained at the high-thigh level are at least 30 mmHg greater than the highest brachial pressure.

▶ Rumwell C, McPharlin M: *Vascular Technology: An Illustrated Review*, 5th edition. Pasadena, Davies Publishing, 2015, p 76.

Q 246

In a normal study, what should the ankle systolic pressure be?

a. less than the highest brachial blood pressure

b. less than the right brachial blood pressure

c. equal to the lowest brachial blood pressure

d. the same as or greater than the highest brachial blood pressure

A 246

D. The same as or greater than the highest brachial blood pressure.

Q 247

In measurements of segmental pressures, gradients of 20–30 mmHg between corresponding segments of the legs indicate:

a. disease below the level in the leg with higher pressure
b. disease above the level in the leg with higher pressure
c. disease at or above the level in the leg with lower pressure
d. no significant disease

A 247

C. Disease at or above the level in the leg with lower pressure.

In addition to pressure gradients between segments on a single limb, horizontal gradients between two limbs at the same level indicate obstructive disease at or above the level in the leg with the lower pressure.

▸ Rumwell C, McPharlin M: *Vascular Technology: An Illustrated Review*, 5th edition. Pasadena, Davies Publishing, 2015, p 75.

Q 248

Following exercise, what is a normal response for ankle pressures in comparison with resting values?

a. no change

b. decrease

c. gradual decrease over 5 minutes

d. increase

A 248

D. Increase.

In a patient without obstructive disease, ankle pressures will increase following exercise. In the presence of arterial obstructive disease, the ankle pressure will decrease immediately after exercise.

▶ Rumwell C, McPharlin M: *Vascular Technology: An Illustrated Review*, 5th edition. Pasadena, Davies Publishing, 2015, pp 77–79.

Q 249

A 57-year-old male presented to the vascular lab for lower extremity arterial testing. Exercise testing was stopped due to symptoms of claudication. Postexercise ankle pressures measured slightly above resting ankle pressures. What is suspected in this patient?

a. occlusion or stenosis at a single level

b. a nonvascular cause of leg pain

c. multilevel arterial disease

d. isolated iliac artery occlusion

A 249

B. A nonvascular cause of leg pain.

If a patient must stop exercising because of leg pain but shows normal ankle pressures, a nonvascular cause of leg pain should be considered.

▶ Rumwell C, McPharlin M: *Vascular Technology: An Illustrated Review*, 5th edition. Pasadena, Davies Publishing, 2015, pp 77–79.

Q 250

An aneurysm resulting from infection is known as:

a. fusiform

b. mycotic

c. saccular

d. ectatic

A 250

B. Mycotic.

Q 251

What does a volume plethysmographic waveform with a normal amplitude, a rounded peak, and an absent dicrotic notch most likely indicate?

a. normal arterial inflow

b. arterial disease proximal to the level of tracing

c. arterial disease distal to the level of tracing

d. arterial occlusion at the level of the tracing

A 251

B. Arterial disease proximal to the level of tracing.

A volume plethysmographic waveform with a flattened systolic peak and absent dicrotic notch is moderately abnormal and always reflects arterial disease proximal to the level of the tracing. Other signs of moderate abnormality include a decrease in the upslope and downslope time that is nearly equal between upslope and downslope.

▸ Rumwell C, McPharlin M: *Vascular Technology: An Illustrated Review*, 5th edition. Pasadena, Davies Publishing, 2015, pp 103–105.

Q 252

How should the patient be positioned to obtain digital pressures of the toes?

a. supine
b. Trendelenburg
c. standing
d. decubitus

A 252

A. Supine.

The patient should be in a supine position while the examiner obtains toe pressures. The head can be elevated 10°–20°.

▶ Rumwell C, McPharlin M: *Vascular Technology: An Illustrated Review*, 5th edition. Pasadena, Davies Publishing, 2015, p 108.

Q 253

A type of plethysmography that detects cutaneous blood flow by sending infrared light into the tissue is termed:

a. photoplethysmography

b. air plethysmography

c. volume plethysmography

d. impedance plethysmography

DAVIES
Registry Reviews & Study Aids

A 253

A. Photoplethysmography.

Photoplethysmography detects cutaneous blood flow by sending infrared light into the tissue with a light-emitting diode. A photodetector receives and measures the reflected infrared light.

- Rumwell C, McPharlin M: *Vascular Technology: An Illustrated Review*, 5th edition. Pasadena, Davies Publishing, 2015, pp 102–114.

Q 254

Following cessation of exercise in an individual with normal vascular function, how long does it take for lower extremity blood flow to return to resting values?

a. 1–5 minutes

b. 5–10 minutes

c. 10–15 minutes

d. as long as 30 minutes

A 254

A. 1–5 minutes.

▸ Strandness DE, Zierler RE: Exercise ankle pressure measurements in arterial disease. In Bernstein EF (ed): *Noninvasive Diagnostic Techniques in Vascular Disease*. St. Louis, Mosby, 1985, pp 575–583.

Q 255

What is the best method for evaluation of a suspected popliteal aneurysm?

a. pulse volume recording
b. duplex ultrasound
c. segmental pressures
d. continuous-wave Doppler

DAVIES
Registry Reviews & Study Aids

A 255

B. Duplex ultrasound.

Q 256

Your patient has undergone a femoral to anterior tibial bypass graft. During routine postoperative surveillance of the graft, you detect retrograde flow in the native anterior tibial artery just proximal to the distal anastomosis. What is the most likely explanation for this finding?

a. It is consistent with severe obstruction in the native outflow artery.

b. It is evident because blood moves from a higher-pressure energy in the bypass graft to the lower-pressure energy of the diseased native vessel.

c. It represents a steal phenomenon that may result in graft failure.

d. It is a normal finding because blood moves from the lower pressure of the bypass to the higher pressure of the diseased native vessel.

A 256

B. It is evident because blood moves from a higher-pressure energy in the bypass graft to the lower-pressure energy of the diseased native vessel.

- Rumwell C, McPharlin M: *Vascular Technology: An Illustrated Review*, 5th edition. Pasadena, Davies Publishing, 2015, p 133.

Q 257

During performance of a postoperative study for a reversed saphenous bypass graft, which of the following potential complications should you consider?

a. stenosis at the proximal anastomosis

b. arteriovenous fistula

c. increased flow secondary to retained valve cusp

d. pseudoaneurysm at mid-graft level

A 257

A. Stenosis at the proximal anastomosis.

▶ Rumwell C, McPharlin M: *Vascular Technology: An Illustrated Review*, 5th edition. Pasadena, Davies Publishing, 2015, p 132.

Q 258

Which of the following is thought normally to occur in stented arteries?

a. increased arterial compliance
b. resected plaque
c. spectral broadening
d. elevated peak systolic velocities

A 258

D. Elevated peak systolic velocities.

▶ Rumwell C, McPharlin M: *Vascular Technology: An Illustrated Review*, 5th edition. Pasadena, Davies Publishing, 2015, p 188.

Q 259

Lower extremity arterial grafts using the great saphenous vein are typically termed either *reversed* or:

a. nonreversed

b. in situ

c. allograft

d. synthetic

A 259

B. In situ.

- Ridgway DP: *Introduction to Vascular Scanning: A Guide for the Complete Beginner*, 4th edition. Pasadena, Davies Publishing, 2014, p 266.

Q 260

Common graft configurations include all **EXCEPT**:

a. fem-fem

b. fem-pop

c. tib-tib

d. ax-fem

A 260

C. Tib-tib.

- Ridgway DP: *Introduction to Vascular Scanning: A Guide for the Complete Beginner*, 4th edition. Pasadena, Davies Publishing, 2014, p 268.

Q 261

In duplex imaging, the best arterial wall image quality is obtained when the beam is at the following angle to the artery walls:

a. 90°

b. 60°

c. 0°

d. oblique

A 261

A. 90°.

The angle of incidence equals the angle of reflectance. Therefore, more echoes return to the transducer with a 90° angle.

▶ Kremkau, Frederick W: *Sonography: Principles and Instruments*, 8th edition. Philadelphia, Elsevier Saunders, 2011, pp 160–161.

Q 262

After catheterization of a cardiac patient, you find a pulsatile mass in the groin. What is the most likely cause?

a. a femoral artery aneurysm

b. a hematoma

c. a pseudoaneurysm of the femoral artery

d. an arteriovenous fistula

A 262

C. A pseudoaneurysm of the femoral artery.

Femoral artery pseudoaneurysms are often found after catheterization. Hematomas after cardiac catheterization are also frequent but usually do not pulsate.

▶ Rumwell CB, McPharlin M: *Vascular Technology: An Illustrated Review*, 5th edition. Pasadena, Davies Publishing, 2015, pp 48–50.

Q 263

Which one of the following changes occurs in the peripheral blood flow of limbs with obstructive arterial disease in response to laboratory-induced ischemia or exercise?

a. Hyperemia is prolonged in obstructed limbs in comparison to limbs with no obstruction.

b. Flow decreases in order to redistribute blood volume to the central circulation.

c. Flow increases more in obstructed limbs than in limbs with no obstruction.

d. Peripheral resistance is increased due to muscle contraction.

A 263

A. Hyperemia is prolonged in obstructed limbs in comparison to limbs with no obstruction.

Hyperemia is prolonged in patients with significant obstruction. Cardiac output is partly a function of how much blood the peripheral circulation is willing to accept. Decreased peripheral resistance, such as after reactive hyperemia or exercise, would tend to increase cardiac output.

- Rumwell C, McPharlin M: *Vascular Technology: An Illustrated Review*, 5th edition. Pasadena, Davies Publishing, 2015, pp 79–80.
- Pellerito JS, Polak JF: *Introduction to Vascular Ultrasonography*, 6th edition. Philadelphia, Elsevier Saunders, 2012, pp 256–257.
- Pellerito JS, Polak JF: *Introduction to Vascular Ultrasonography*, 7th edition. Philadelphia, Elsevier Saunders, 2020.

Q 264

What is the difference between the protocols for cardiac treadmill testing and claudication treadmill testing?

a. A single, faster speed is used for cardiac testing.
b. The patient is closely monitored by technologists during cardiac testing.
c. Speed is varied during cardiac testing.
d. Elevation is varied during claudication testing.

A 264

C. Speed is varied during cardiac testing.

The standard cardiac treadmill protocol aims to increase the heart rate to a specific target level by increasing the speed and elevation of the treadmill at specific time intervals during the examination. Treadmill testing for claudication generally uses one unvarying speed and elevation. Both types of exam include blood pressure monitoring, as well as observation by technologists. There is some cardiac risk associated with claudication testing.

▶ Rumwell CB, McPharlin M: *Vascular Technology: An Illustrated Review*, 5th edition. Pasadena, Davies Publishing, 2015, pp 77–78.

Q 265

You obtain the following segmental pressure readings from your patient: right brachial = 144 mmHg, left brachial = 140 mmHg, right high thigh = 110 mmHg, left high thigh = 164 mmHg. These findings would **NOT** result from:

a. right common femoral obstruction

b. right common iliac obstruction

c. right external iliac obstruction

d. aortoiliac obstruction

DAVIES Registry Reviews & Study Aids

A 265

D. Aortoiliac obstruction.

Since the left high-thigh pressure is within normal limits, the aortic segment cannot be included in the diagnosis of obstruction.

Q 266

How would you describe the velocities measured in a reversed saphenous vein bypass graft?

a. lower proximally and higher distally
b. greater than 100 cm/sec throughout the graft
c. the same throughout the graft
d. higher proximally and lower distally

A 266

D. Higher proximally and lower distally.

The velocities will vary depending on the inflow, size of graft, location (and quality) of valve cusps, presence of stenoses, and tightness of distal anastomosis. Generally the velocities in a reversed vein graft will be lower distally (compared to proximally) because of the increased size of the graft distally.

Q 267

The "kissing stent" angioplasty/stent technique is useful for:

a. the adductor canal region

b. total occlusions

c. infrarenal arteries only

d. bifurcations

A 267

D. Bifurcations.

This is a method of deploying balloon angioplasty and arranging stents at bifurcations, avoiding occlusion of one branch while dilating the other. The technique can be used anywhere, including coronary arteries.

▸ Schneider PA, Rutherford RB: Endovascular interventions in the management of chronic lower extremity ischemia. In Rutherford RB (ed): *Vascular Surgery*, 5th edition. Philadelphia, Saunders, 2000, p 1048.

Q 268

During ultrasound-guided compression of a pseudoaneurysm, you know to observe all of the following points of technique **EXCEPT**:

a. Use color flow to monitor flow in the common femoral artery.
b. Use color flow to confirm that flow remains biphasic within the pseudoaneurysm.
c. Use color flow to confirm that flow is obliterated in the pseudoaneurysm.
d. Release pressure for a short time at 10- to 15-minute intervals.

A 268

B. Use color flow to confirm that flow remains biphasic within the pseudo-aneurysm.

Ultrasound-guided thrombin injection is increasingly becoming the gold standard for pseudoaneurysm therapy, although manual compression remains a standard treatment option.

- Dzijan-Horn M, Langwieser N, Groha P, et al: Coronary interventions: safety and efficacy of a potential treatment algorithm by using manual compression repair and ultrasound-guided thrombin injection for the management of iatrogenic femoral artery pseudoaneurysm in a large patient cohort. Circulation 7:207–215, 2014.
- Pellerito JS, Polak JF: *Introduction to Vascular Ultrasonography*, 6th edition. Philadelphia, Elsevier Saunders, 2012, pp 331–334.
- Pellerito JS, Polak JF: *Introduction to Vascular Ultrasonography*, 7th edition. Philadelphia, Elsevier Saunders, 2020.

Q 269

The incidence of pseudoaneurysms is:

a. staying the same
b. decreasing
c. increasing
d. not associated with iatrogenic causes

A 269

C. Increasing.

As the number of transluminal procedures increases, we are seeing more iatrogenic pseudoaneurysms.

▶ Schwartz LB, Clark ET, Gewertz BL: Anastomotic and other pseudoaneurysms. In Rutherford RB (ed): *Vascular Surgery*, 5th edition. Philadelphia, Saunders, 2000, p 753.

Q 270

This waveform profile is characteristic of which of the following?

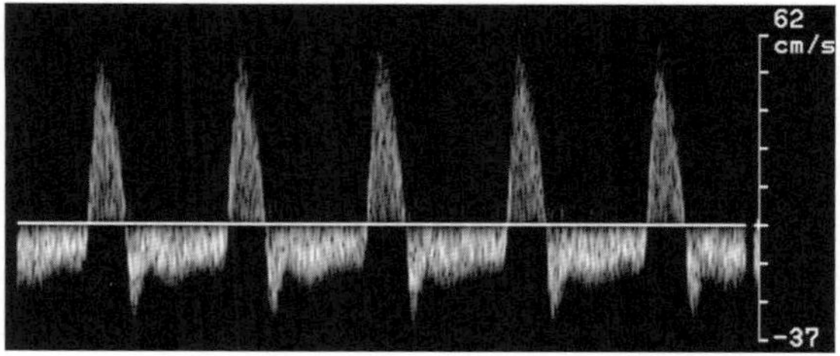

a. neck of pseudoaneurysm

b. arteriovenous communication

c. dampened signal obtained proximal to arterial occlusion

d. hyperemic flow

A 270

A. Neck of pseudoaneurysm.

Q 271

These segmental pressure measurements were obtained from a 67-year-old male with symptoms of claudication. What values are used to determine the ABI?

Right	Segment	Left
160 mmHg	brachial	172 mmHg
189 mmHg	high thigh	150 mmHg
161 mmHg	above knee	126 mmHg
157 mmHg	below knee	104 mmHg
118 mmHg	ankle	84 mmHg

a. right 118/160, left 84/172

b. right 118/172, left 84/172

c. right 118/160, left 84/160

d. right 118/172, left 84/160

A 271

B. Right 118/172, left 84/172.

The right ABI = 0.68 and the left ABI = 0.48.

The ankle/brachial index is calculated by dividing the ankle pressure by the higher of the two brachial pressures.

▶ Rumwell C, McPharlin M: *Vascular Technology: An Illustrated Review*, 5th edition. Pasadena, Davies Publishing, 2015, pp 74–75.

Q 272

A 72-year-old female is referred to the vascular lab for evaluation of right lower extremity claudication. Bilateral brachial blood pressures are 135 mmHg and bilateral ankle pressures are 300 mmHg. This is most likely related to:

a. severe hypertension

b. cuff artifact due to improper size

c. incompressible arteries due to arterial calcification

d. misalignment of cuff on the extremity

A 272

C. Incompressible arteries due to arterial calcification.

Q 273

A 58-year-old male presents to the vascular lab with an abdominal bruit and bilateral weak lower extremity pulses. Review these segmental pressures and determine the level of disease.

Right	Segment	Left
155 mmHg	brachial	148 mmHg
101 mmHg	high thigh	100 mmHg
98 mmHg	above knee	98 mmHg
69 mmHg	below knee	89 mmHg
87 mmHg	ankle	88 mmHg

a. right deep femoral artery, left popliteal

b. aortoiliac disease

c. right superficial femoral artery, obstruction, left popliteal artery obstruction

d. bilateral trifurcation disease

A 273

B. Aortoiliac disease.

Q 274

Determine the ABIs from the segmental pressure study in question 273.

a. right 0.56, left 0.59

b. right 0.56, left 0.56

c. right 0.59, left 0.56

d. right 1.78, left 1.68

A 274

B. Right 0.56, left 0.56.

Q 275

What test is used to detect arterial patency of the palmar arch?

a. photoplethysmography

b. reactive hyperemia

c. Allen test

d. thoracic outlet evaluation

A 275

C. Allen test.

▶ Rumwell C, McPharlin M: *Vascular Technology: An Illustrated Review*, 5th edition. Pasadena, Davies Publishing, 2015, pp 84–87.

Q 276

From which artery is a Doppler tracing at the medial malleolus obtained?

a. dorsalis pedis
b. peroneal
c. posterior tibial
d. anterior tibial

A 276

C. Posterior tibial.

Q 277

A loss of the triphasic waveform in the popliteal artery can result from:

a. distal vasodilatation
b. proximal occlusion
c. exercise
d. all of the above

A 277

D. All of the above.

Q 278

A dampened waveform demonstrating a delayed acceleration time is obtained in the common femoral artery. What is the most likely reason for this finding?

a. distal occlusion

b. pseudoaneurysm

c. inflow disease

d. exercise

A 278

C. Inflow disease.

▶ Rumwell C, McPharlin M: *Vascular Technology: An Illustrated Review*, 5th edition. Pasadena, Davies Publishing, 2015, p 68.

Q 279

How should the patient be positioned to allow segmental pressures of the lower extremity to be obtained?

a. reverse Trendelenburg

b. supine with the extremities at the same level as the heart

c. Trendelenburg

d. supine with the extremities below the level of the heart

DAVIES
Registry Reviews & Study Aids

A 279

B. Supine with the extremities at the same level as the heart.

▶ Rumwell C, McPharlin M: *Vascular Technology: An Illustrated Review*, 5th edition. Pasadena, Davies Publishing, 2015, p 71.

Q 280

Which ABI is indicative of rest pain?

a. > 1.0

b. 0.9–1.0

c. 0.5–0.9

d. < 0.5

A 280

D. < 0.5.

Q 281

Evaluate the segmental pressures presented here. What is the most likely reason for the horizontal difference of 28 mmHg at the level below the knee?

Right	Segment	Left
150 mmHg	brachial	151 mmHg
189 mmHg	high thigh	192 mmHg
178 mmHg	above knee	173 mmHg
134 mmHg	below knee	162 mmHg
97 mmHg	ankle	152 mmHg

a. right inflow disease

b. cuff artifact

c. left femoral artery disease

d. right popliteal and tibial vessel disease

A 281

D. Right popliteal and tibial vessel disease.

Q 282

A great toe pressure of 30 mmHg or less indicates:

a. a good chance of healing for foot or toe ulcer
b. normality
c. arterial calcification due to diabetes
d. a poor chance of healing for foot or toe ulcer

A 282

D. A poor chance of healing for foot or toe ulcer.

Great toe pressures are especially useful for evaluating diabetic patients, in whom ankle pressures are unreliable because of arterial calcification. The normal great toe pressure is 60 mmHg. When great toe pressures are 30 mmHg or less, foot and toe ulcerations are unlikely to heal.

▶ Rumwell C, McPharlin M: *Vascular Technology: An Illustrated Review*, 5th edition. Pasadena, Davies Publishing, 2015, p 77.

Q 283

Which of the following is **NOT** a contraindication for treadmill stress testing?

a. history of cardiac problems
b. history of claudication
c. history of stroke
d. shortness of breath

A 283

B. History of claudication.

Exercise testing is used to help differentiate between true claudication and neurogenic claudication and to help determine the presence or absence of collaterals. It is indicated when resting measurements are not grossly abnormal and/or symptoms do not correlate with the resting measurements. Contraindications to exercise stress testing include shortness of breath, hypertension, cardiac problems, stroke, and walking problems.

▶ Rumwell C, McPharlin M: *Vascular Technology: An Illustrated Review*, 5th edition. Pasadena, Davies Publishing, 2015, p 77.

Q 284

A stenosis of the superficial femoral artery showed a peak systolic velocity of 180 cm/sec and a prestenotic velocity of 85 cm/sec. What percentage diameter stenosis is suggested by these values?

a. ≥25%

b. ≥50%

c. ≥75%

d. ≥90%

A 284

B. ≥50%.

In duplex evaluation of the lower extremity arterial circulation, a ratio is calculated between the prestenotic systolic velocity and the peak systolic velocity within the stenosis. A 2:1 ratio suggests a greater than 50% diameter stenosis, and a 4:1 ratio suggests a greater than 75% diameter stenosis.

▸ Rumwell C, McPharlin M: *Vascular Technology: An Illustrated Review*, 5th edition. Pasadena, Davies Publishing, 2015, p 133.

Q 285

In reactive hyperemia testing, the blood pressure cuffs are inflated to suprasystolic pressure levels for how long?

a. 45 seconds

b. 1–2 minutes

c. 3–5 minutes

d. 8 minutes

A 285

C. 3–5 minutes.

Reactive hyperemia testing is an alternative to exercise testing for stressing the peripheral arterial system. This test is very uncomfortable for the patient. The blood pressure cuff is inflated above the highest brachial blood pressure for 3–5 minutes. Ischemia and vasodilatation occur distal to the cuff. Once the cuff is released, the changes in ankle pressure are similar to those obtained after exercise, although a transient decrease in pressure of 17%–34% may be seen in normal limbs with reactive hyperemia.

▸ Rumwell C, McPharlin M: *Vascular Technology: An Illustrated Review*, 5th edition. Pasadena, Davies Publishing, 2015, pp 79–80.

Q 286

How would you characterize retrograde flow in the native artery at the site of distal anastomosis of a lower extremity?

a. an early indication of graft failure

b. indicative of arteriovenous fistula

c. a normal finding

d. diagnostic of distal occlusive disease

DAVIES
Registry Reviews & Study Aids

A 286

C. A normal finding.

Blood flow always courses in a direction from high pressure to low pressure. In this case, there is higher pressure within the normal graft and lower pressure within the native artery. This commonly results in some blood coursing up the native artery (retrograde) at the site of the distal anastomosis. This retrograde flow perfuses tissue above the level of the anastomotic site and provides additional benefit to the patient.

▶ Rumwell C, McPharlin M: *Vascular Technology: An Illustrated Review*, 5th edition. Pasadena, Davies Publishing, 2015, p 132.

Q 287

All of the following statements regarding arteriography are true **EXCEPT**:

a. It requires an intra-arterial injection.
b. It gives anatomic information regarding the vascular system.
c. It employs a liquid contrast agent to image the arterial lumen.
d. It gives functional information regarding the vascular system.

DAVIES Registry Reviews & Study Aids

A 287

D. This statement–"It gives functional information regarding the vascular system"–is **NOT** true. Arteriography gives anatomic but not functional (physiologic) information.

▶ Rumwell C, McPharlin M: *Vascular Technology: An Illustrated Review*, 5th edition. Pasadena, Davies Publishing, 2015, pp 173–175.

Q 288

How is vasospasm demonstrated arteriographically?

a. as a severe narrowing of the arterial lumen
b. as having a "string of beads" appearance
c. as a vibrating artery
d. Vasospasm cannot be detected arteriographically.

A 288

A. As a severe narrowing of the arterial lumen.

Rumwell C, McPharlin M: *Vascular Technology: An Illustrated Review*, 5th edition. Pasadena, Davies Publishing, 2015, p 177.

Q 289

Arteriography is contraindicated in a patient with:

a. renal failure

b. diabetes

c. malignancy

d. vascular disease

A 289

A. Renal failure.

- Rumwell C, McPharlin M: *Vascular Technology: An Illustrated Review*, 5th edition. Pasadena, Davies Publishing, 2015, p 174.

Q 290

What is the most common cause of portal hypertension in the United States?

a. schistosomiasis
b. hyperlipidemia
c. cirrhosis
d. hypertension

A 290

C. Cirrhosis.

Q 291

You have received a request to evaluate blood flow within the splanchnic arteries. Which of the following groups of blood vessels should you examine?

a. main portal vein, right portal vein, left portal vein

b. right and left renal arteries and veins

c. right and left common iliac and external iliac arteries

d. celiac artery, superior mesenteric artery, inferior mesenteric artery

DAVIES Registry Reviews & Study Aids

A 291

D. Celiac artery, superior mesenteric artery, inferior mesenteric artery.

The splanchnic arteries are the vessels that supply blood to the gut. These primarily are the celiac artery, superior mesenteric artery (SMA), and inferior mesenteric artery (IMA). Stenosis or occlusion involving these vessels can result in chronic ischemia of the bowel, known as mesenteric ischemia.

Q 292

You are performing a Doppler exam on a patient with suspected renovascular hypertension. Which diagnostic parameter is the best indicator of renovascular disease?

a. renal/aortic ratio

b. A/B ratio

c. systolic/diastolic ratio

d. pulsatility index

A 292

A. Renal/aortic ratio.

Renovascular hypertension is caused by renal artery stenosis. Stenosis of the renal artery can be determined by obtaining a renal/aortic ratio (RAR). This is a ratio of the highest velocity obtained in the renal artery to the normal velocity of the aorta obtained at the level of the renal artery origins. A ratio of ≥ 3.5 is considered by most to indicate a significant renal artery stenosis. This would mean that the velocity in the renal artery is 3.5 times faster than the velocity in the aorta.

- Rumwell C, McPharlin M: *Vascular Technology: An Illustrated Review*, 5th edition. Pasadena, Davies Publishing, 2015, pp 142–149.
- Granata F, Fiorini S, Andrulli F, et al: Doppler ultrasound and renal artery stenosis: an overview. J Ultrasound Med Biol 12:133–143, 2009.

Q 293

Which abdominal vessel is most commonly compromised by compression of the median arcuate ligament of the diaphragm?

a. celiac artery

b. inferior vena cava

c. left gastric artery

d. superior mesenteric artery

DAVIES
Registry Reviews & Study Aids

A 293

A. Celiac artery.

The median arcuate ligament of the diaphragm crosses the anterior aspect of the aorta slightly above (i.e., superior to) the celiac artery (also known as the celiac trunk). In some patients, during expiration, this anatomic situation can lead to compression of the celiac artery and high velocities. The abnormally high velocities are present during expiration but return to normal during inspiration. These patients may present with an abdominal bruit.

Q 294

The following are common features of renal allograft rejection **EXCEPT**:

a. increased allograft size

b. increased cortical echogenicity

c. decreased flow resistance in parenchymal arteries

d. increased prominence of the renal pyramids

A 294

C. Decreased flow resistance in parenchymal arteries.

In renal allograft rejection the flow resistance in the parenchymal arteries tends to increase. This will be manifested as a decrease in diastolic flow. Normal flow in the parenchymal arteries of a renal allograft is low-resistance with forward flow throughout the cardiac cycle. A decrease, absence, or reversal of flow in diastole is indicative of rejection.

▸ Rumwell C, McPharlin M: *Vascular Technology: An Illustrated Review*, 5th edition. Pasadena, Davies Publishing, 2015, pp 155–157.

Q 295

Which of the following would be most likely to occur as a result of increased portal venous pressure in a patient with portal hypertension?

a. enlarged coronary vein
b. aortic dissection
c. hepatic artery aneurysm
d. cavernous transformation

A 295

A. Enlarged coronary vein.

The coronary vein normally drains into the splenic vein. With portal hypertension, the increased portal venous pressure decreases flow into the portal system. Consequently, vessels that normally drain into the portal system become enlarged and often find alternate routes of flow. The coronary vein may reverse its flow direction and feed into esophageal varices. These can break down, causing life-threatening bleeding episodes. Cavernous transformation may occur in patients with portal hypertension, but only in the presence of portal vein thrombosis and recanalization. Cavernous transformation of the portal vein most commonly occurs when the liver is normal. Most patients with portal hypertension have underlying liver cirrhosis. Aortic dissection and hepatic artery aneurysm are not associated with portal hypertension.

Q 296

The most common location of atherosclerotic disease of the renal artery is:

a. mid

b. distal

c. intrarenal

d. proximal

DAVIES
Registry Reviews & Study Aids

A 296

D. Proximal.

Atherosclerotic disease tends to affect the bifurcations of arteries. The renal artery is most commonly affected at its origin from the aorta. This is considered to be the proximal portion of the vessel. Fibromuscular disease more commonly affects the mid to distal aspect of the renal artery.

Q 297

You are performing a Doppler study on a patient with fibromuscular dysplasia. Which of the following conditions is most commonly associated with this abnormality?

a. mesenteric ischemia

b. portal hypertension

c. renovascular hypertension

d. Budd-Chiari syndrome

A 297

C. Renovascular hypertension.

Fibromuscular hyperplasia is a condition in which the artery has a series of small dilatations and narrowings that create the angiographic appearance of a string of beads or pearls. In contrast to atherosclerosis, fibromuscular hyperplasia tends to affect younger individuals and is more common in women than men. It can affect the renal arteries and tends to be located in the mid to distal end of the vessel. The splanchnic vessels are not commonly affected.

Q 298

Budd-Chiari syndrome is a cause of portal hypertension resulting from:

a. hepatic vein obstruction
b. inferior mesenteric vein thrombus
c. hepatic artery stenosis
d. superior vena cava thrombus

A 298

A. Hepatic vein obstruction.

Hepatic vein obstruction leaves no way for portal venous hepatic arterial blood to be removed. Therefore hepatic congestion occurs, resulting in ascites, progressive hepatic dysfunction, and portal hypertension. In its acute form the disease is rapidly fatal unless treated surgically. Liver tumors are a separate possible cause of hepatic vein obstruction.

▸ Johansen KH, Helton WS, Rikkers LF: Operative therapy for portal hypertension. In Rutherford RB (ed): *Vascular Surgery*, 5th edition. Philadelphia, Saunders, 2000, p 1578.

Q 299

A patient presents to the vascular lab with an abdominal bruit, weight loss, and postprandial pain. Obstruction of which vessel is most likely responsible for these symptoms?

a. renal artery
b. portal vein
c. superior mesenteric artery
d. splenic vein

A 299

C. Superior mesenteric artery.

Chronic mesenteric ischemia may result from obstruction of the arteries that supply the gut. The primary vessel supplying the intestine is the superior mesenteric artery. The inferior mesenteric artery and celiac trunk may also contribute. Symptoms usually do not occur unless two of these three arteries are obstructed. A rich collateral network exists between these three vessels, making chronic mesenteric ischemia a rare disorder.

- Rumwell C, McPharlin M: *Vascular Technology: An Illustrated Review*, 5th edition. Pasadena, Davies Publishing, 2015, pp 149–154.
- Baxter BT, Pearce WH: Diagnosis and surgical management of chronic mesenteric ischemia. In Strandness DE, van Breda A (eds): *Vascular Diseases: Surgical and Interventional Therapy*. New York, Churchill Livingstone, 1994, pp 795–802.

Q 300

What does retrograde flow in an enlarged coronary vein suggest?

a. inferior vena cava thrombus

b. renal vein thrombus

c. iliac vein thrombus

d. portal hypertension

A 300

D. Portal hypertension.

▶ Rumwell C, McPharlin M: *Vascular Technology: An Illustrated Review*, 5th edition. Pasadena, Davies Publishing, 2015, pp 155, 288, 329, 351–352.

Q 301

The paraumbilical vein drains into a network of varices that can be seen on the abdomen radiating from the umbilicus. These varices are known as:

a. caput medusae

b. cavernous transformation

c. veins of Sappey

d. azygos veins

A 301

A. Caput medusae.

Q 302

The abdominal aorta is considered aneurysmal when it reaches or exceeds a diameter of:

a. 3 cm

b. 4 cm

c. 5 cm

d. 6 cm

A 302

A. 3 cm.

▶ Ridgway DP: *Introduction to Vascular Scanning: A Guide for the Complete Beginner*, 4th edition. Pasadena, Davies Publishing, 2014, p 102.

Q 303

This Doppler waveform was obtained from a segmental artery within the kidney in a patient with severe hypertension. Which diagnosis is most likely?

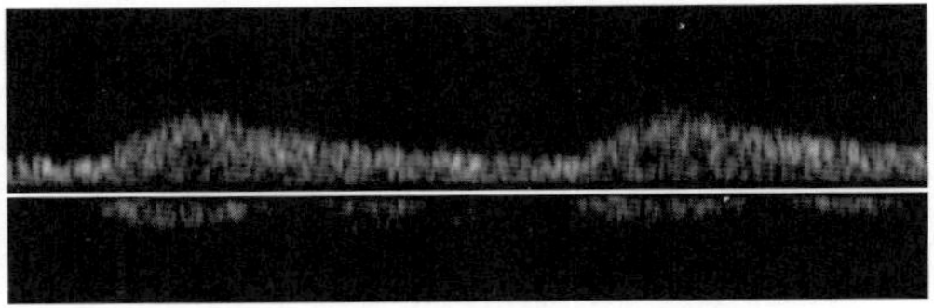

a. presence of parenchymal renal disease

b. ipsilateral renal vein thrombosis

c. presence of ipsilateral main renal artery stenosis

d. renal failure

DAVIES
Registry Reviews & Study Aids

A 303

C. Presence of ipsilateral main renal artery stenosis.

The delayed systolic upstroke and absence of early systolic peak in the waveform of this segmental renal artery indicates proximal stenosis of greater than 60 percent or occlusion in the main renal artery. This waveform shape is termed *tardus parvus*, a term that literally means "late and weak."

- Rumwell C, McPharlin M: *Vascular Technology: An Illustrated Review*, 5th edition. Pasadena, Davies Publishing, 2015, p 148.
- Stavros T, Harshfield D: Renal Doppler, renal artery stenosis, and renovascular hypertension: direct and indirect duplex sonographic abnormalities in patients with renal artery stenosis. Ultrasound Quarterly 12:217–263, 1994.

Q 304

This waveform can be described as:

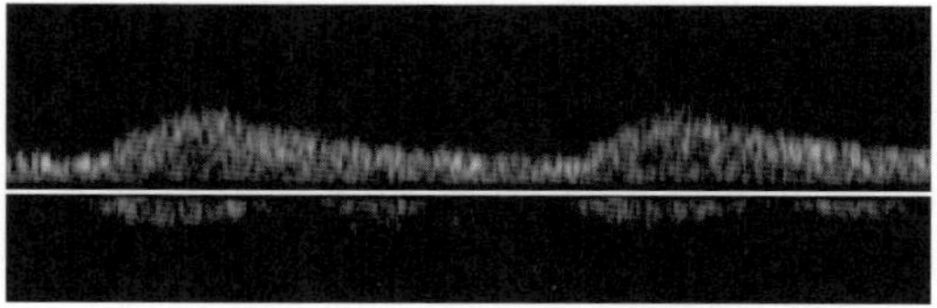

a. triphasic

b. monophasic

c. multiphasic

d. biphasic

A 304

B. Monophasic.

Q 305

Both of these waveforms were obtained from segmental renal arteries in the renal hilum. Which waveform shows a normal resistance to flow?

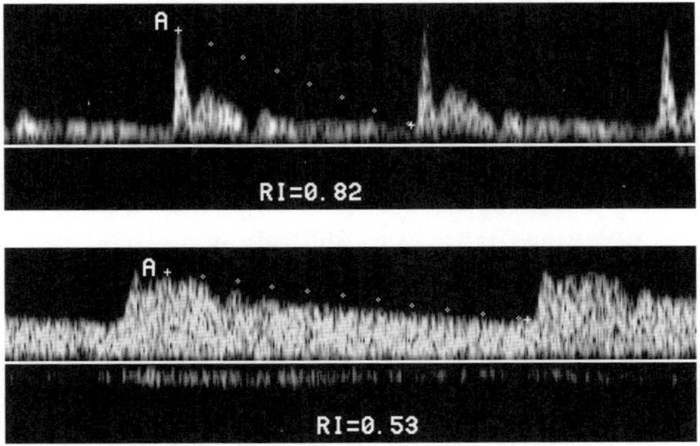

a. top

b. bottom

A 305

B. Bottom.

The normal RI (resistive index) in the kidney is less than 0.7. As the RI increases, the amount of diastolic flow will decrease. Normal waveforms obtained from the main renal artery or from arteries within the kidney are of low resistance with forward flow throughout the cardiac cycle. Increased resistance may be seen in cases of renal disease, renal vein thrombosis, and a hematoma or other mass pressing on the kidney.

- Rumwell C, McPharlin M: *Vascular Technology: An Illustrated Review*, 5th edition. Pasadena, Davies Publishing, 2015, pp 147–148.
- Stavros T, Harshfield D: Renal Doppler, renal artery stenosis, and renovascular hypertension: direct and indirect duplex sonographic abnormalities in patients with renal artery stenosis. Ultrasound Quarterly 12:217–263, 1994.

Q 306

What pathology is most likely responsible for this abnormal waveform?

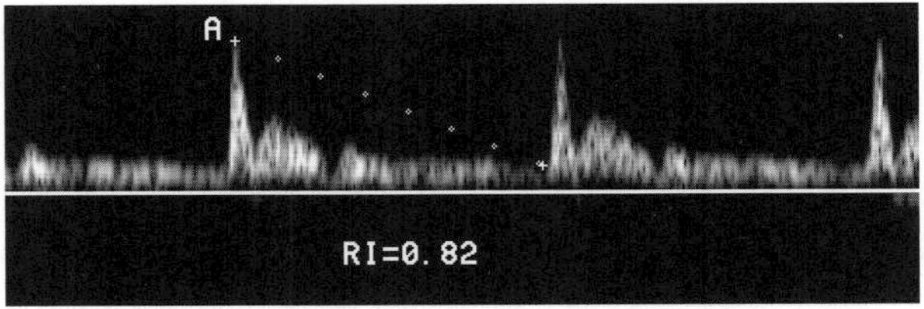

a. renal artery stenosis

b. parenchymal renal disease

c. renal artery fibromuscular dysplasia

d. renal artery arteriovenous fistula

A 306

B. Parenchymal renal disease.

Q 307

Under which of the following conditions will you see increased diastolic flow in the superior mesenteric artery?

a. postprandial state

b. stenosis

c. replaced hepatic artery

d. all of the above

DAVIES Registry Reviews & Study Aids

A 307

D. All of the above.

The superior mesenteric artery (SMA) will show low-resistance flow in the postprandial state, when stenosis is present, or when variant anatomy such as a replaced hepatic artery arises from the proximal SMA.

Q 308

Which of the following arteries will **NOT** demonstrate low-resistance waveforms in the fasting state?

a. hepatic artery
b. splenic artery
c. renal artery
d. inferior mesenteric artery

DAVIES
Registry Reviews & Study Aids

A 308

D. Inferior mesenteric artery.

Arteries that feed parenchymal organs–including the celiac, hepatic, splenic, and renal arteries in the abdomen–demonstrate low-resistance waveforms with forward flow present throughout the entire cardiac cycle. The superior and inferior mesenteric arteries show little diastolic flow in the fasting state. Following a meal, the diastolic flow in the superior mesenteric artery increases to as much as three times its fasting level.

- Rumwell C, McPharlin M: *Vascular Technology: An Illustrated Review*, 5th edition. Pasadena, Davies Publishing, 2015, p 145.
- Baxter BT, Pearce WH: Diagnosis and surgical management of chronic mesenteric ischemia. In Strandness DE, van Breda A (eds): *Vascular Diseases: Surgical and Interventional Therapy*. New York, Churchill Livingstone, 1994, pp 795–802.

Q 309

What is the most common anatomic location of renal allografts?

a. left iliac fossa

b. right iliac fossa

c. mid pelvis

d. Morison's pouch

A 309

B. Right iliac fossa.

Most renal allografts (transplants) are located in the right lower quadrant.

▸ Rumwell C, McPharlin M: *Vascular Technology: An Illustrated Review*, 5th edition. Pasadena, Davies Publishing, 2015, pp 154–155.

Q 310

Which vessel is most commonly involved in the median arcuate ligament syndrome?

a. superior mesenteric artery

b. portal vein

c. inferior mesenteric artery

d. celiac trunk

DAVIES
Registry Reviews & Study Aids

A 310

D. Celiac trunk.

The median arcuate ligament syndrome usually involves only the celiac trunk, although rarely it may also cause compression of the superior mesenteric artery.

- Matsumoto AH, Muehle C, Casada D, et al: Compression of the superior mesenteric artery by the median arcuate ligament: a cause for mesenteric ischemia. Vascular Surgery 28:489–493, 1994.

Q 311

Direct Doppler interrogation of the renal arteries is limited by:

a. stenosis in accessory renal arteries, which may not be detected
b. the difficulty of obtaining Doppler angles less than 60° at the renal artery origins
c. patient body habitus, which can limit access to the renal arteries
d. all of the above

A 311

D. All of the above.

There are two methods for detecting renal artery stenosis with Doppler ultrasound, a direct and an indirect method. The direct method involves Doppler interrogation throughout the length of each renal artery. Limitations of the technique include the high incidence of multiple renal arteries (in as many as 25% of patients), difficulty obtaining adequate Doppler angles to the renal artery origins, and difficulty completely visualizing the renal arteries due to bowel gas or patient body habitus. When multiple renal arteries are present, they are frequently difficult to visualize sonographically. The indirect technique involves Doppler interrogation of the segmental or interlobar arteries within the kidney. This indirect evaluation overcomes the limitations of poor patient body habitus and inadequate Doppler angles. The presence of multiple renal arteries is not a problem with this technique since Doppler samplings are taken from the upper, mid, and lower poles of the kidney. Limitations of the indirect technique include the inability to distinguish between stenosis and total occlusion and the inability to detect stenoses of less than 60% diameter reduction.

▸ Stavros T, Harshfield D: Renal Doppler, renal artery stenosis, and renovascular hypertension: direct and indirect duplex sonographic abnormalities in patients with renal artery stenosis. Ultrasound Quarterly 12:217–263, 1994.

Q 312

A 53-year-old male presents to the vascular lab with a six-month history of severe hypertension and abdominal bruit. Which vessel is most likely the source of the patient's symptoms?

a. superior mesenteric artery

b. celiac trunk

c. hepatic artery

d. renal artery

A 312

D. Renal artery.

Q 313

A patient is referred to rule out Budd-Chiari syndrome. Which vessel would be imaged?

a. innominate vein

b. common femoral vein

c. hepatic vein

d. internal jugular vein

A 313

C. Hepatic vein.

Q 314

Which waveform (top or bottom) represents abnormal portal vein flow?

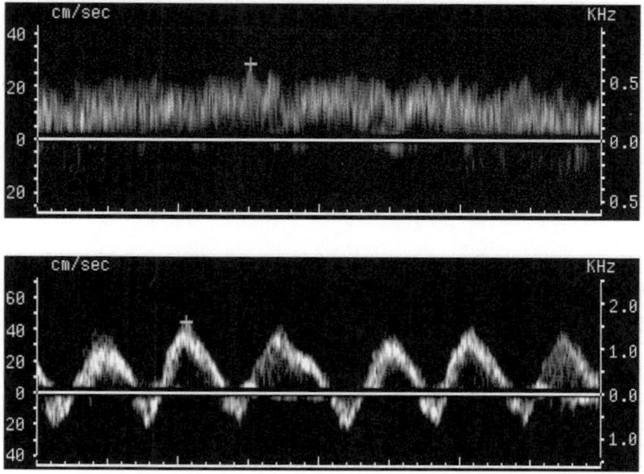

a. top

b. bottom

Abdominal and Visceral / Testing and Treatment / AIT—Hotspot

A 314

B. Bottom.

The normal waveform obtained from the portal vein is a mildly undulating signal. Prominent pulsatility or bidirectional flow as seen in the bottom waveform is an abnormal finding and can be indicative of right heart failure, tricuspid regurgitation, portal vein–hepatic artery fistula, portal hypertension, and other abnormalities.

- Rumwell C, McPharlin M: *Vascular Technology: An Illustrated Review*, 5th edition. Pasadena, Davies Publishing, 2015, pp 280, 288, 319, 321–322.
- Rosenthal SJ, Harrison LA, Baxter KG, et al: Doppler US of helical flow in the portal vein. RadioGraphics 15:1103–1111, 1995.

Q 315

What might this abnormal portal venous waveform indicate?

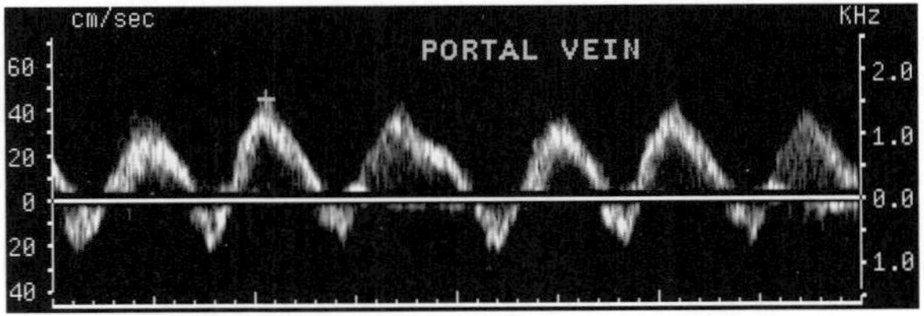

a. hepatic metastases

b. tricuspid regurgitation

c. hepatic artery thrombosis

d. hepatic infarction

DAVIES
Registry Reviews & Study Aids

A 315

B. Tricuspid regurgitation.

A pulsatile portal vein waveform can result from right heart failure, tricuspid regurgitation, portal vein–hepatic artery fistula, portal hypertension, and other abnormalities.

▸ Rosenthal SJ, Harrison LA, Baxter KG, et al: Doppler US of helical flow in the portal vein. RadioGraphics 15:1103–1111, 1995.

Q 316

Following a transjugular intrahepatic portosystemic shunt (TIPS) procedure, which of these findings is normal?

a. hepatofugal flow in the main portal vein

b. hepatofugal flow in the splenic vein

c. hepatofugal flow in intrahepatic portal radicles

d. all of the above

DAVIES
Registry Reviews & Study Aids

A 316

C. Hepatofugal flow in intrahepatic portal radicles.

Hepatofugal flow in the intrahepatic portal vein branches is a common finding following successful TIPS because flow follows the path of least resistance. Scarring in the liver due to cirrhosis results in high resistance to flow through intrahepatic portal branches. The TIPS stent produces a path of low resistance so flow in the portal branches reverses and courses toward the stent.

Q 317

During the Valsalva maneuver, what happens to pressure in the abdomen and thorax?

a. intrathoracic pressure increases, abdominal pressure increases

b. intrathoracic pressure decreases, abdominal pressure decreases

c. intrathoracic pressure increases, abdominal pressure decreases

d. intrathoracic pressure decreases, abdominal pressure increases

A 317

A. Intrathoracic pressure increases, abdominal pressure increases.

▶ Rumwell C, McPharlin M: *Vascular Technology: An Illustrated Review*, 5th edition. Pasadena, Davies Publishing, 2015, p 280.

Q 318

During inspiration, what happens to pressure in the abdomen and thorax?

a. Intrathoracic pressure increases, abdominal pressure increases.
b. Intrathoracic pressure increases, abdominal pressure decreases.
c. Intrathoracic pressure decreases, abdominal pressure decreases.
d. Intrathoracic pressure decreases, abdominal pressure increases.

DAVIES
Registry Reviews & Study Aids

A 318

D. Intrathoracic pressure decreases, abdominal pressure increases.

- Rumwell C, McPharlin M: *Vascular Technology: An Illustrated Review*, 5th edition. Pasadena, Davies Publishing, 2015, p 280.

Q 319

A 57-year-old female with a history of long-term alcohol abuse is referred for a portal venous duplex exam. The main portal vein cannot be identified at the porta hepatis, but instead multiple channels with hepatopetal flow are seen. This is consistent with:

a. caput medusae

b. paraumbilical flow

c. cavernous transformation

d. portal-hepatic fistula

A 319

C. Cavernous transformation.

In cases of portal vein thrombosis, recanalization may occur, producing an appearance of multiple channels of hepatopetal flow within the porta hepatis instead of one main portal vein. This is termed *cavernous transformation of the portal vein.*

Q 320

All **EXCEPT** which of the following findings are associated with portal hypertension?

a. splenomegaly

b. gallbladder wall varices

c. ascites

d. lymphadenopathy

A 320

D. Lymphadenopathy.

Lymphadenopathy is not associated with portal hypertension. Splenomegaly is almost always present in cases of portal hypertension. Gallbladder wall varices are a less common feature but have a clear association. Ascites is frequently present and should increase suspicion for the presence of portal vein thrombosis.

Q 321

A patient in a hypercoagulable state is seen to have thrombosis of the right renal vein by duplex sonography. What other findings may be seen in association with this?

a. thrombus within the inferior vena cava

b. decreased diastolic flow in the right renal artery

c. poor visualization of interlobular flow by color Doppler

d. all of the above

A 321

D. All of the above.

Q 322

How would you describe the normal waveform of the renal vein?

a. phasic with respiration

b. highly pulsatile

c. flat and continuous

d. triphasic

A 322

A. Phasic with respiration.

Q 323

A spontaneous splenorenal shunt is an abnormal connection between the splenic and left renal veins and is associated with:

a. renovascular hypertension

b. portal hypertension

c. renal failure

d. renal cell carcinoma

DAVIES
Registry Reviews & Study Aids

A 323

B. Portal hypertension.

Q 324

The term *endoleak* refers to:

a. a Baker's cyst

b. a lesion with intraplaque hemorrhage

c. blood flow into an abdominal aortic aneurysmal sac following placement of an endograft

d. an arteriovenous fistula

A 324

C. Blood flow into an abdominal aortic aneurysmal sac following placement of an endograft.

An endograft is a stent that is placed to exclude an abdominal aortic aneurysm from the systemic circulation, thereby reducing the size of the aneurysmal sac and eliminating blood flow within it. If flow is detected within the sac following this procedure, or if the sac fails to shrink or grows larger, suspect an endoleak. See also the answer to question 325.

- Rumwell C, McPharlin M: *Vascular Technology: An Illustrated Review*, 5th edition. Pasadena, Davies Publishing, 2015, pp 188–192.
- Ridgway DP: *Introduction to Vascular Scanning: A Guide for the Complete Beginner*, 4th edition. Pasadena, Davies Publishing, 2014, p 102.

Q 325

Your patient has undergone placement of an aortic stent graft to exclude an abdominal aortic aneurysm. His latest surveillance study documented one of the more commonly occurring endoleaks, related to a lumbar artery. What type of endoleak is this?

a. type I

b. type II

c. type III

d. type IV

A 325

B. Type II.

Following stent graft repair for an abdominal aortic aneurysm, an endoleak may have occurred if blood flow is observed in the sac or if the size of the sac fails to diminish or grows larger. Several types have been identified:

- Type I: An attachment endoleak at proximal and/or distal attachment site(s), considered one of the most dangerous and in need of repair.
- Type II: A branch leak originating from a native vessel that normally branches off the aorta. Branches include the lumbar artery and the inferior mesenteric artery (IMA). This leak allows retrograde flow into the residual aneurysmal sac with resulting blood flow outside or around the endograft that keeps the sac pressurized. Type II leaks are often watched rather than immediately repaired, although they will likely be repaired if expansion of the anerusymal sac is observed.
- Type III: A leak from the connections of modular components, or "modular connect" leak. This type of leak is also considered one of the most dangerous and should be repaired.
- Type IV: A transgraft endoleak, resulting from minute tears in the fabric or changes in wall porosity. Advances in graft construction have virtually eliminated this type of endoleak.

▶ Rumwell C, McPharlin M: *Vascular Technology: An Illustrated Review*, 5th edition. Pasadena, Davies Publishing, 2015, pp 189–190.

Q 326

Which of the following is a normal finding in a patient who has a transjugular intrahepatic portosystemic shunt (TIPS)?

a. hepatofugal flow in the main portal vein
b. hepatopetal flow in the main portal vein
c. absence of flow in the portal vein
d. hepatofugal flow in the splenic vein

A 326

B. Hepatopetal flow in the main portal vein.

Flow should be hepatopetal: toward the liver. Hepatofugal flow, away from the liver, is an abnormal finding in both the portal and splenic veins. No flow is bad too.

- Rumwell C, McPharlin M: *Vascular Technology: An Illustrated Review*, 5th edition. Pasadena, Davies Publishing, 2015, pp 155, 274, 319–320.
- Pellerito JS, Polak JF: *Introduction to Vascular Ultrasonography*, 6th edition. Philadelphia, Elsevier Saunders, 2012, p 512.
- Pellerito JS, Polak JF: *Introduction to Vascular Ultrasonography*, 7th edition. Philadelphia, Elsevier Saunders, 2020.

Q 327

Patient preparation for abdominal scanning typically includes:

a. avoiding carbonated drinks

b. avoiding cigarettes and gum

c. fasting for 6–12 hours before the study

d. all of the above

A 327

D. All of the above.

▶ Ridgway DP: *Introduction to Vascular Scanning: A Guide for the Complete Beginner*, 4th edition. Pasadena, Davies Publishing, 2014, p 106.

Q 328

Which of the following is the purpose of intravascular ultrasound (IVUS)?

a. to ascertain where a stent should be placed
b. to determine whether a stent is properly deployed during angioplasty
c. to diagnose thrombus in the coronary arteries
d. all of the above

A 328

D. All of the above.

▶ Rumwell C, McPharlin M: *Vascular Technology: An Illustrated Review*, 5th edition. Pasadena, Davies Publishing, 2015, pp 184–185.

Q 329

For saphenous vein mapping, which transducer would be the best choice?

a. 3 MHz curved array
b. 4–6 MHz curved array
c. 5 MHz linear array
d. 7–10 MHz linear array

A 329

D. 7–10 MHz linear array.

Q 330

You are mapping the saphenous veins in a patient scheduled for coronary artery bypass surgery. You have discovered that the saphenous veins are inadequate for harvesting. Which of the following veins would be best to evaluate as an alternate graft?

a. deep femoral vein

b. cephalic vein

c. popliteal vein

d. axillary vein

DAVIES
Registry Reviews & Study Aids

A 330

B. Cephalic vein.

The cephalic or basilic vein may be mapped as a possible conduit for bypass surgery when the great or small saphenous vein is too small, diseased, or absent. Deep veins such as the deep femoral, popliteal, or axillary vein are not used.

Q 331

You have been asked to perform a vein mapping of the saphenous vein. Which of the following techniques would be most helpful?

a. Decrease the room temperature so the small saphenous vein will become dilated.

b. Use a high-frequency probe and light probe pressure to track the saphenous vein.

c. Place the patient in an upright position to improve visualization of the saphenous vein.

d. Place the patient in a prone position to improve access to the saphenous vein.

A 331

B. Use a high-frequency probe and light probe pressure to track the saphenous vein.

The highest-frequency linear array probe available should be used to track the saphenous vein because it is very superficial. Very light probe pressure should be used since it is easy to compress the vein by resting the probe on the skin. When the vein cannot be visualized, decreasing probe pressure will often help to demonstrate the vein. If the room temperature is too cold, the veins will be small and hard to see. The patient should be placed in a supine position with the leg externally rotated and the knee slightly bent.

▶ Talbot SR: Venous imaging technique. In Talbot SR, Oliver MA: *Techniques of Venous Imaging*. Pasadena, Davies Publishing, 1992, pp 59–118.

Q 332

A patient presents with a pseudoaneurysm following arterial puncture. For ultrasound-guided compression of the pseudoaneurysm, how long would each compression last before you check for cessation of flow into the pseudoaneurysm?

a. 1 minute

b. 30 minutes

c. 10 minutes

d. 45 minutes

A 332

C. 10 minutes.

Repair of a pseudoaneurysm by ultrasound-guided compression is accomplished by applying pressure with the ultrasound transducer over the neck of the pseudoaneurysm. Pressure is increased until a cessation of flow is apparent within the pseudoaneurysm while maintaining flow within the native artery. Multiple compressions lasting approximately 10 minutes each are usually necessary to obliterate the flow within the pseudoaneurysm and its communicating channel.

- Rumwell C, McPharlin M: *Vascular Technology: An Illustrated Review*, 5th edition. Pasadena, Davies Publishing, 2015, p 195.
- Hertz SM, Brener BJ: Ultrasound-guided pseudoaneurysm compression: efficacy after coronary stenting and angioplasty. J Vasc Surg 26:913–918, 1997.

Q 333

Arteriovenous fistula is a complication that most commonly occurs with:

a. angioplasty
b. reversed vein bypass grafts
c. atherectomy
d. in situ grafts

A 333

D. In situ grafts.

Arteriovenous fistula is not a complication of reversed vein bypass grafts, atherectomy, or angioplasty. It is a complication of in situ bypass grafts. Arteriovenous fistulas occur when one of the venous branches of the saphenous vein is not ligated, resulting in communication between the graft and an adjacent vein.

Arteriovenous fistulas may also be congenital, traumatic, surgically created for hemodialysis, and so forth.

- Rumwell C, McPharlin M: *Vascular Technology: An Illustrated Review*, 5th edition. Pasadena, Davies Publishing, 2015, p 132.
- Polak JF: Arterial sonography: efficacy for the diagnosis of arterial disease of the lower extremity. AJR 161:235–243, 1993.

Q 334

The type of aneurysm related to arterial trauma that results in blood escaping through a defect in the vessel wall and extravasating into the surrounding tissue is a:

a. pseudoaneurysm

b. fusiform aneurysm

c. saccular aneurysm

d. dissecting aneurysm

A 334

A. Pseudoaneurysm.

▶ Rumwell C, McPharlin M: *Vascular Technology: An Illustrated Review*, 5th edition. Pasadena, Davies Publishing, 2015, p 49.

Q 335

A patient presents with swelling around the puncture site of arteriography. Duplex sonography reveals a high-velocity tract from the artery leading to a large hematoma. What is the term for this pathology?

a. dissection

b. pseudoaneurysm

c. arteriovenous fistula

d. subintimal hematoma

DAVIES
Registry Reviews & Study Aids

A 335

B. Pseudoaneurysm.

Q 336

Which of the following describes a typical venous Doppler waveform obtained proximal to an arteriovenous fistula?

a. increased velocity and pulsatility

b. prominent respiratory phasicity

c. unchanged from normal

d. continuous low velocity

A 336

A. Increased velocity and pulsatility.

Q 337

What characteristics would be demonstrated by a typical arterial Doppler waveform obtained proximal to an arteriovenous fistula?

a. triphasic
b. high resistance with no diastolic flow
c. low resistance with increased flow
d. bidirectional with increased velocities during systole and reverse flow in diastole

A 337

C. Low resistance with increased flow.

Q 338

Which statement regarding an arteriovenous fistula is **NOT** true?

a. A fistula located close to the heart increases the potential for cardiac failure.

b. Arterial flow proximal to the fistula is markedly increased.

c. Blood pressure in the distal artery is always increased.

d. A thrill may be felt over the fistula site.

DAVIES
Registry Reviews & Study Aids

A 338

C. This statement–"blood pressure in the distal artery is always increased"–is **NOT** true.

The blood pressure in the distal artery is always decreased in the presence of an arteriovenous fistula.

▶ Rumwell C, McPharlin M: *Vascular Technology: An Illustrated Review*, 5th edition. Pasadena, Davies Publishing, 2015, pp 165–167.

Q 339

Which of the following describes the classic flow pattern in the neck of a traumatic pseudoaneurysm?

a. high-velocity antegrade flow in systole with retrograde flow in diastole
b. high resistance with absence of flow in diastole
c. low resistance with high-velocity flow during systole
d. trickle flow

A 339

A. High-velocity antegrade flow in systole with retrograde flow in diastole.

The classic flow pattern in the neck of a pseudoaneurysm is bidirectional. Since blood tends to flow from high pressure to low pressure, it flows into the pseudoaneurysm in systole and back into the native artery during diastole.

Q 340

Your patient has undergone cardiac catheterization. Ultrasonographic findings in the lower extremity include low-resistance, high-velocity flow in the common femoral artery and pulsatile flow in the common femoral vein. A prominent bruit is present. These findings are most closely associated with:

a. pseudoaneurysm

b. arterial dissection

c. traumatic arteriovenous fistula

d. arterial and venous compression due to hematoma

A 340

C. Traumatic arteriovenous fistula.

Arteriovenous fistula is an abnormal direct connection between an artery and vein. Fistulas may occur as complications of arterial puncture. When a fistula is present, arterial flow will be preferentially shunted into the low-pressure venous system. This will cause pulsatility in the downstream component of the affected vein. Since much of the arterial flow is coursing directly into the low-resistance venous system, increased diastolic flow and high velocities will be seen in the artery proximal to the fistula.

Q 341

A Brescia-Cimino fistula is a type of:

a. traumatic fistula

b. dialysis access anastomosis

c. surgical correction for thoracic outlet syndrome

d. congenital fistula

A 341

B. Dialysis access anastomosis.

This arteriovenous fistula between the radial artery and the cephalic vein is the preferred permanent vascular access for hemodialysis due to its fewer complications and greater longevity compared to other types of accesses.

- Rumwell C, McPharlin M: *Vascular Technology: An Illustrated Review*, 5th edition. Pasadena, Davies Publishing, 2015, p 122.
- Finlay DI, Longley DG, Foshager MC, et al: Duplex and color Doppler sonography of hemodialysis arteriovenous fistulas and grafts. RadioGraphics 13:983–999,1993.

Q 342

This waveform is a typical example of the Doppler signal obtained from a(n):

a. pseudoaneurysm neck
b. lower extremity arterial bypass graft
c. dialysis access graft
d. aneurysmal artery

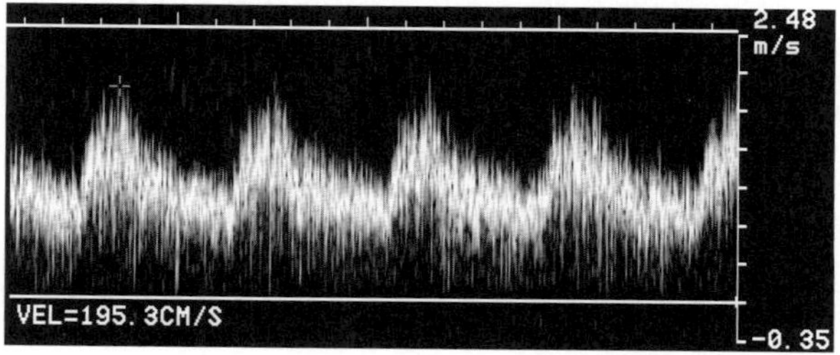

DAVIES
Registry Reviews & Study Aids

A 342

C. Dialysis access graft.

Because a dialysis graft forms a direct fistula between an artery and a vein, the arterial signal will have high diastolic velocities reflecting the low resistance in the draining vein. Typical systolic velocities range between 100 and 400 cm/sec.

Q 343

Which is a complication of dialysis access grafts?

a. arterial steal

b. aneurysm

c. venous stenosis

d. all of the above

A 343

D. All of the above.

Complications of dialysis access grafts include arterial and venous stenoses, graft thrombosis, infection, aneurysm, pseudoaneurysm formation, arterial steal, and hematoma.

▶ Finlay DI, Longley DG, Foshager MC, et al: Duplex and color Doppler sonography of hemodialysis arteriovenous fistulas and grafts. RadioGraphics 13:983–999,1993.

Q 344

In liver transplants, what is the location of the arterial anastomosis of the native common hepatic artery to the donor hepatic artery?

a. in the posterior aspect of the right lobe of the liver

b. in the medial segment of the left lobe of the liver

c. at the porta hepatis where the hepatic artery enters the liver

d. several centimeters proximal to the hepatic hilum

A 344

D. Several centimeters proximal to the hepatic hilum.

▶ Foley WD: *Color Doppler Flow Imaging*. Boston, Andover Medical Publishers, 1991.

Q 345

The Doppler frequency most likely to be used to evaluate the penile artery is:

a. 2 MHz

b. 4 MHz

c. 20 MHz

d. 7 MHz

A 345

D. 7 MHz.

▶ Rumwell C, McPharlin M: *Vascular Technology: An Illustrated Review*, 5th edition. Pasadena, Davies Publishing, 2015, p 95.

Q 346

Which of the following represents a normal penile/brachial index (PBI)?

a. 0.75 or greater
b. 0.65–0.74
c. less than 0.65
d. All are normal.

A 346

A. 0.75 or greater.

A normal PBI is 0.75 or greater. The calculation is based on the highest brachial pressure.

▶ Rumwell C, McPharlin M: *Vascular Technology: An Illustrated Review*, 5th edition. Pasadena, Davies Publishing, 2015, p 95.

Q 347

What is an advantage of using the radial artery instead of the great or small saphenous vein for coronary artery bypass grafts?

a. vessel caliber similar to that of coronary arteries
b. thicker vessel wall
c. longer patency rates
d. all of the above

A 347

D. All of the above.

All of these are potential advantages of using the radial artery over the saphenous vein for coronary artery bypass grafts. An additional advantage is that many patients do not have adequate saphenous veins for harvesting due to prior thrombus, small size, or prior use.

- Ridgway DP: *Introduction to Vascular Scanning: A Guide for the Complete Beginner*, 4th edition. Pasadena, Davies Publishing, 2014, pp 274, 290.
- Winkler J, Lohr J, Bukhari RH, et al: Evaluation of the radial artery for use in coronary artery bypass grafting. J Vasc Technol 22:23–29, 1998.

Q 348

The internal thoracic artery is a branch of which of the following arteries?

a. innominate
b. vertebral
c. subclavian
d. axillary

DAVIES
Registry Reviews & Study Aids

A 348

C. Subclavian.

Q 349

Which of the following is a common feature of temporal arteritis?

a. dissection
b. aneurysm
c. intimal thickening
d. tortuosity
e. ectasia

A 349

C. Intimal thickening.

Temporal arteritis causes marked thickening of the intima. It may be localized, focal, or widespread. Patients tend to present with severe headache. Other symptoms may include scalp tenderness, visual disturbance, joint pain, and painful chewing. Blindness can occur as a result of ischemic optic neuropathy in less than 20% of patients.

▶ Beers MH, Berkow R (eds): *The Merck Manual*, 17th ed. Whitehouse Station, NJ, Merck.

Q 350

Which of the following describes the Adson maneuver used in diagnosis of thoracic outlet syndrome?

a. The patient hyperabducts the arm in conjunction with rapid opening and closing of the hand.

b. The patient sits straight and crosses the arms in front during deep inspiration.

c. The patient assumes a military posture with the shoulders braced down.

d. The patient's arm is at a 90° angle to the torso with the head turned toward the affected side and then away from the affected side during deep inspiration.

A 350

D. The patient's arm is at a 90° angle to the torso with the head turned toward the affected side and then away from the affected side during deep inspiration.

Q 351

Symptoms associated with thoracic outlet syndrome include all of the following **EXCEPT**:

a. increased blood pressure on the affected side

b. aching of shoulder and forearm

c. numbness or tingling of the arm

d. increased discomfort with upward arm positions

A 351

A. Increased blood pressure on the affected side.

Q 352

Which of the following would **NOT** be associated with arterial trauma?

a. fibromuscular dysplasia

b. hematoma

c. pseudoaneurysm

d. dissection

A 352

A. Fibromuscular dysplasia.

Fibromuscular dysplasia is a condition in which a series of small dilatations and narrowings occur in an artery, creating an angiographic pattern referred to as a "string of pearls" or "string of beads." It is more commonly seen in females and young individuals but is not associated with arterial trauma. Dissection results from an intimal tear in an artery and may be caused by trauma or other factors such as fibromuscular dysplasia, hypertension, and Marfan syndrome. A hematoma is simply a swelling caused by a mass of blood (usually clotted) resulting from a tear in a blood vessel. A pseudoaneurysm may also be a result of arterial trauma. It occurs when there is a tear in a vessel with blood leaking out into a space that is not confined by the vessel wall. An arterial track with bidirectional flow is seen leading from the artery to the pulsing hematoma.

▶ Rumwell C, McPharlin M: *Vascular Technology: An Illustrated Review*, 5th edition. Pasadena, Davies Publishing, 2015, pp 177, 215–216, 255.

Q 353

You are performing a Doppler exam on a 32-year-old female who was recently involved in a car accident. She received a blow to the left side of her body. She presents with an abdominal bruit, back pain, and hypertension. Which of the following conditions is most likely?

a. Takayasu's arteritis involving the abdominal aorta

b. fibromuscular dysplasia involving the splenic and common hepatic arteries

c. dissection involving the abdominal aorta and possibly the renal arteries

d. inflammatory aneurysm of the infrarenal abdominal aorta

A 353

C. Dissection involving the abdominal aorta and possibly the renal arteries.

Of the conditions listed, only arterial dissection is related to trauma. Dissection of the abdominal aorta can compromise flow to the renal arteries, resulting in hypertension. Dissection may even extend into the renal arteries and compromise flow.

Q 354

You are performing an ultrasound exam on a patient with a gunshot wound involving the posterior tibial artery. What artifact is associated with metallic objects such as bullets?

a. enhancement

b. multipath

c. comet-tail

d. mirror-image

A 354

C. Comet-tail.

Comet-tail artifacts are associated with metallic objects such as bullets or surgical clips. The appearance of a comet-tail artifact is a series of bands underneath the metallic object. The artifact is caused by multiple reverberations of the sound wave within the tiny metallic structure.

Q 355

You are trying to determine whether to map the great saphenous vein for use as a lower extremity bypass graft. Which of the following observations would render the vein suitable for this purpose?

a. Vein measures 3.0 mm × 3.2 mm.

b. Diameter of the vessel is unchanged following application of a proximal tourniquet.

c. Vessel walls do not coapt.

d. Mural calcifications are present.

DAVIES
Registry Reviews & Study Aids

A 355

A. Vein measures 3.0 mm $\times$ 3.2 mm.

▸ Rumwell C, McPharlin M: *Vascular Technology: An Illustrated Review*, 5th edition. Pasadena, Davies Publishing, 2015, p 64.

Q 356

PTFE, often used for dialysis grafts, has the following sonographic appearance:

a. fuzzy
b. double-walled
c. essentially the same as veins
d. very bright, with acoustic shadowing

A 356

B. Double-walled.

See also question 469.

▶ Ridgway DP: *Introduction to Vascular Scanning: A Guide for the Complete Beginner*, 4th edition. Pasadena, Davies Publishing, 2014, p 267.

Q 357

The Brescia-Cimino fistula is a common configuration for dialysis access because of the:

a. large radius of the brachial veins
b. proximity of the basilic vein and ulnar artery
c. proximity of the brachial artery and basilic vein
d. proximity of the cephalic vein and radial artery

A 357

D. Proximity of the cephalic vein and radial artery.

- Ridgway DP: *Introduction to Vascular Scanning: A Guide for the Complete Beginner*, 4th edition. Pasadena, Davies Publishing, 2014, p 301.

Q 358

An abnormal flow rate for a radial artery/cephalic vein dialysis fistula is:

a. less than 200 ml/min
b. 400 to 900 ml/min
c. 1000 to 1500 ml/min
d. greater than 1500 ml/min

A 358

A. Less than 200 ml/min.

A flow rate of around 300 ml/min is required for dialysis.

- Pellerito JS, Polak JF: *Introduction to Vascular Ultrasonography*, 6th edition. Philadelphia, Elsevier Saunders, 2012, pp 287–289.
- Pellerito JS, Polak JF: *Introduction to Vascular Ultrasonography*, 7th edition. Philadelphia, Elsevier Saunders, 2020.

Q 359

The digital/brachial systolic pressure ratio in an extremity with a dialysis fistula:

a. is greater than 1.00
b. is less than 0.80
c. is less than 0.50
d. should not be measured

DAVIES
Registry Reviews & Study Aids

A 359

D. Should not be measured.

In an extremity with a dialysis fistula, you should avoid measuring brachial blood pressure. You could measure the contralateral brachial blood pressure.

Q 360

In duplex assessment of dialysis fistulas (synthetic or native), common abnormalities include all **EXCEPT**:

a. stenosis at the venous anastomosis

b. high flow rates exceeding 300 ml/min

c. false aneurysm caused by needle puncture

d. aneurysm of the graft

A 360

B. High flow rates exceeding 300 ml/min.

The fistula should have fairly high flow rates to allow for dialysis. The other answer choices are possible abnormalities to look for when scanning.

▸ Ridgway DP: *Introduction to Vascular Scanning: A Guide for the Complete Beginner*, 4th edition. Pasadena, Davies Publishing, 2014, p 301.

Q 361

Complications associated with hemodialysis access grafts include all of the following **EXCEPT**:

a. distal limb ischemia
b. decreased distal venous pressure
c. pseudoaneurysm
d. congestive heart failure

A 361

B. Decreased distal venous pressure.

With hemodialysis access grafts, distal venous hypertension (not hypotension) may develop as a complication due to reversal of flow in the distal vein away from the fistula.

Q 362

The common format for archiving and outputting medical images is:

a. PACS

b. CDROM

c. DICOM

d. MEDCOM

DAVIES Registry Reviews & Study Aids

A 362

C. DICOM.

DICOM stands for Digital Imaging and Communications in Medicine; this is the most common form of medical image storage now in use. It allows for storage and also for digital transfer on networks.

▶ Ridgway DP: *Introduction to Vascular Scanning: A Guide for the Complete Beginner*, 4th edition. Pasadena, Davies Publishing, 2014, p 69.

Q 363

What is PACS?

a. a common name for lower-frequency probes

b. a control for gain at different depths

c. the stage of image processing involving compression

d. a digital storage and retrieval system

A 363

D. A digital storage and retrieval system.

PACS stands for Picture Archiving and Communication System.

▶ Ridgway DP: *Introduction to Vascular Scanning: A Guide for the Complete Beginner*, 4th edition. Pasadena, Davies Publishing, 2014, p 69.

Q 364

Which of these actions would be most in keeping with the ALARA principle during vascular interrogation?

a. Complete the diagnostic scan using the lowest output power that is reasonably achievable.

b. Prolong the exam to allow the patient to communicate symptoms he/she is feeling during the exam.

c. Maximize the acoustic output to shorten the duration of the exam.

d. Allow multiple students to scan a patient for training purposes.

A 364

A. Complete the diagnostic scan using the lowest output power that is reasonably achievable.

ALARA stands for "as low as reasonably achievable."

Q 365

All of the following should be discussed with patients undergoing an ultrasound-guided intraoperative procedure examination **EXCEPT**:

a. probable diagnoses

b. what to wear to the procedure

c. how to position themselves during the procedure

d. aftercare measures

A 365

A. Probable diagnoses.

Q 366

What should patients understand prior to undergoing a vascular ultrasound examination?

a. Ultrasound is uncomfortable but well tolerated.

b. The gel applied to the patient's skin during the procedure will help the patient relax.

c. Ultrasound does not expose the patient to ionizing radiation.

d. The patient should be sure to void urine prior to the procedure.

A 366

C. Ultrasound does not expose the patient to ionizing radiation.

Q 367

Which of the following must you do to comply with HIPAA requirements?

a. Avoid conversations with patients.
b. Store patient information so it is accessible to all physicians and staff.
c. Store files in a locked vault or safe after the examination.
d. Remove notations that identify a patient in an image used for publication.

A 367

D. Remove notations that identify a patient in an image used for publication.

Q 368

What is the significance of the Occupational Safety and Health Administration (OSHA) in the noninvasive testing environment?

a. It provides guidance for testing protocols.

b. It is concerned primarily with patient safety.

c. It oversees regulations ensuring a safe environment for workers.

d. It regulates compliance with standards related to the Health Insurance Portability and Accountability Act of 1996 (HIPAA).

DAVIES Registry Reviews & Study Aids

A 368

C. It oversees regulations ensuring a safe environment for workers.

▶ Rumwell C, McPharlin M: *Vascular Technology: An Illustrated Review*, 5th edition. Pasadena, Davies Publishing, 2015, p 367.

Q 369

What is the term for the ability of a noninvasive test to detect disease when it is present?

a. negative predictive value

b. specificity

c. accuracy

d. sensitivity

A 369

D. Sensitivity.

Calculation: True positives ÷ (True positives + False negatives).

▶ Rumwell C, McPharlin M: *Vascular Technology: An Illustrated Review*, 5th edition. Pasadena, Davies Publishing, 2015, p 358.

Q 370

What is the term for the ability of a noninvasive test to identify that no disease is present when there is no disease?

a. negative predictive value

b. specificity

c. accuracy

d. sensitivity

DAVIES
Registry Reviews & Study Aids

A 370

B. Specificity.

Calculation: True negatives ÷ (True negatives + False positives).

▶ Rumwell C, McPharlin M: *Vascular Technology: An Illustrated Review*, 5th edition. Pasadena, Davies Publishing, 2015, p 358.

Q 371

Which of the following is calculated by dividing the total number of correct tests by the total number of all tests?

a. negative predictive value

b. specificity

c. accuracy

d. sensitivity

A 371

C. Accuracy.

Accuracy is the percentage of correct diagnoses made by the noninvasive test.

▶ Rumwell C, McPharlin M: *Vascular Technology: An Illustrated Review*, 5th edition. Pasadena, Davies Publishing, 2015, p 358.

Q 372

The number of true positives divided by the number of true positives + false positives describes which of the following?

a. sensitivity

b. positive predictive value

c. accuracy

d. specificity

A 372

B. Positive predictive value.

The positive predictive value describes the percentage of individuals with a positive noninvasive test result who actually have the disease.

▶ Rumwell C, McPharlin M: *Vascular Technology: An Illustrated Review*, 5th edition. Pasadena, Davies Publishing, 2015, p 358.

Q 373

What is the term for the proportion of test results that correctly predict normality?

a. accuracy
b. sensitivity
c. specificity
d. negative predictive value

A 373

D. Negative predictive value.

Calculation: True negatives ÷ (True negatives + False negatives).

▸ Rumwell C, McPharlin M: *Vascular Technology: An Illustrated Review*, 5th edition. Pasadena, Davies Publishing, 2015, p 358.

Q 374

If the noninvasive test results were positive but the gold standard showed normal results, how would you refer to the noninvasive test results?

a. false negative

b. false positive

c. true positive

d. true negative

A 374

B. False positive.

A false-positive test is one in which the noninvasive test results were positive but the gold standard test results were negative (i.e., normal).

▸ Rumwell C, McPharlin M: *Vascular Technology: An Illustrated Review*, 5th edition. Pasadena, Davies Publishing, 2015, pp 359–362.

Q 375

What is the best way to prepare a transducer for intraoperative use?

a. autoclave it

b. immerse it for 72 hours in Cidex solution

c. clean it with soap and water

d. place the transducer and acoustic gel within a sterile sleeve or bag

A 375

D. Place the transducer and acoustic gel within a sterile sleeve or bag.

Autoclaving a transducer will destroy its piezoelectric properties.

Q 376

According to Poiseuille's law, what would occur to the pressure gradient across an arterial segment in which the radius has been reduced by ½?

a. no effect

b. decrease

c. There is not enough information to determine the effect.

d. increase

A 376

D. Increase.

Q 377

The tendency of objects to maintain their status quo is called:

a. hydrostatic pressure

b. kinetic energy

c. potential energy

d. inertia

A 377

D. Inertia.

Q 378

Where would you obtain a dampened Doppler signal?

a. A

b. B

c. C

d. none of the above

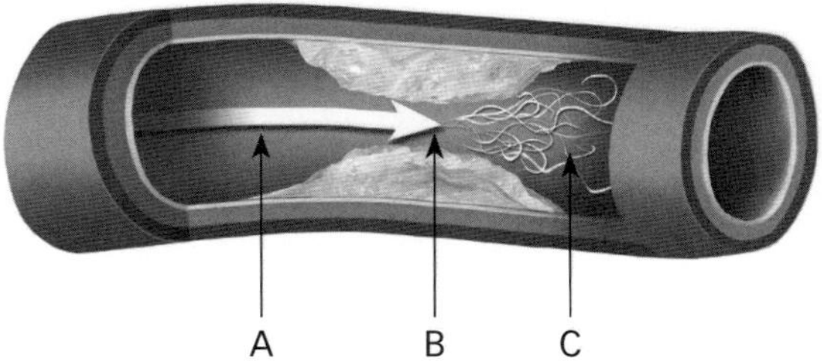

A 378

A. A.

▶ Rumwell C, McPharlin M: *Vascular Technology: An Illustrated Review*, 5th edition. Pasadena, Davies Publishing, 2015, pp 25–26.

Q 379

Where would you obtain a Doppler signal that shows spectral broadening?

a. A

b. B

c. C

d. none of the above

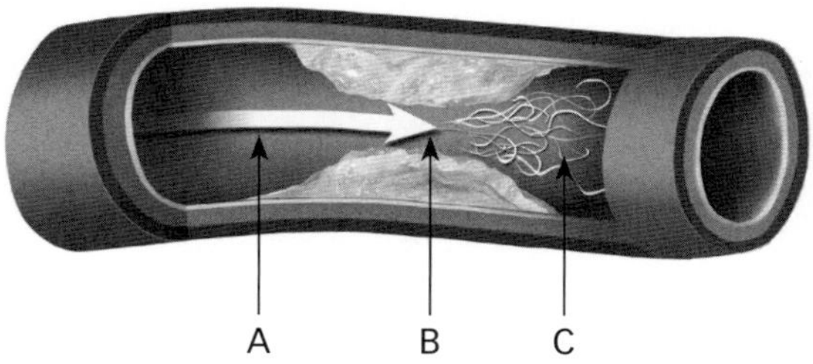

A 379

C. C.

▶ Rumwell C, McPharlin M: *Vascular Technology: An Illustrated Review*, 5th edition. Pasadena, Davies Publishing, 2015, pp 25–26, 39–41.

Q 380

Where would you find the lowest pressure?

a. A

b. B

c. C

d. none of the above

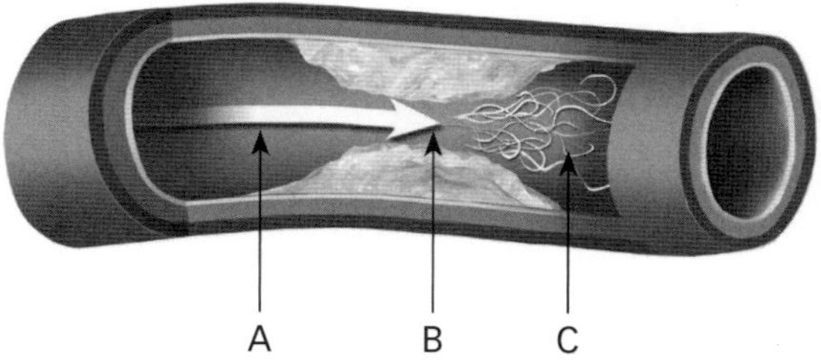

Physiology and Fluid Dynamics / Arterial Hemodynamics / AIT—Hotspot

DAVIES
Registry Reviews & Study Aids

A 380

B. B.

- Rumwell C, McPharlin M: *Vascular Technology: An Illustrated Review*, 5th edition. Pasadena, Davies Publishing, 2015, pp 25–26, 39–41.
- Kremkau FW: *Doppler Ultrasound*. Philadelphia, Saunders, 1990.

Q 381

Where would the Reynolds number be greatest?

a. A

b. B

c. C

d. none of the above

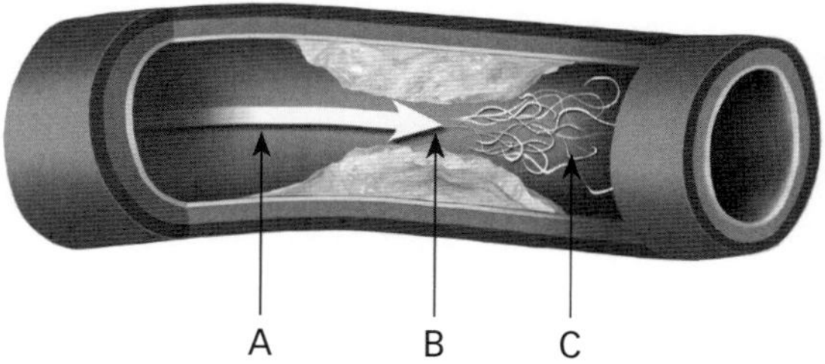

A 381

C. C.

▶ Rumwell C, McPharlin M: *Vascular Technology: An Illustrated Review*, 5th edition. Pasadena, Davies Publishing, 2015, pp 24–26.

Q 382

Where would the Doppler signal show the highest bandwidth?

a. A

b. B

c. C

d. none of the above

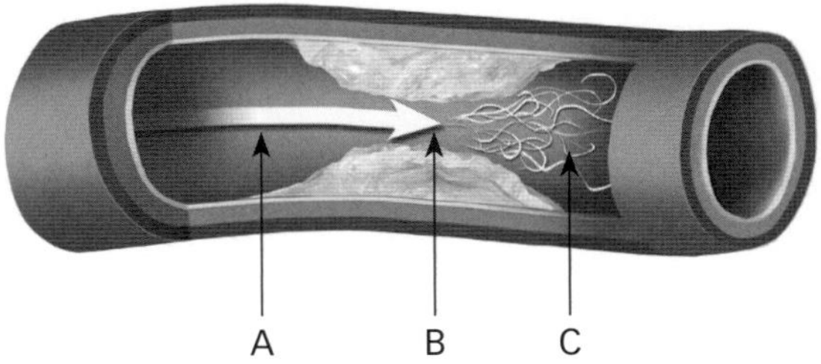

DAVIES
Registry Reviews & Study Aids

A 382

C. C.

Q 383

Where would you find laminar flow?

a. A

b. B

c. C

d. none of the above

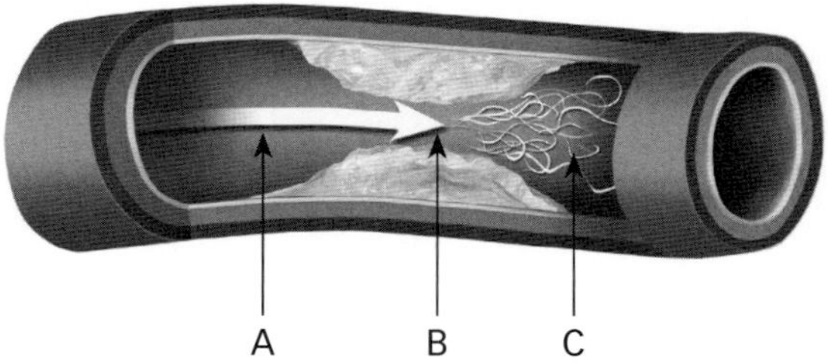

A 383

D. None of the above.

Q 384

What term best describes the pulse profile in this illustration?

a. blunt

b. parabolic

c. laminar

d. flat

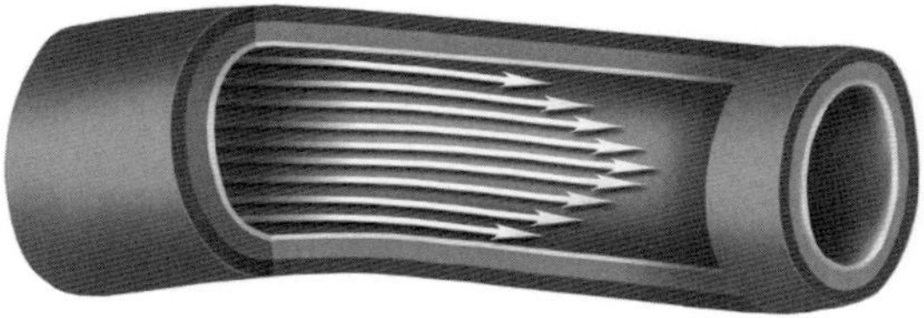

A 384

B. Parabolic.

Q 385

The resistance to flow offered by the fluid in motion is termed:

a. viscosity
b. pressure gradient
c. kinetic energy
d. inertia

A 385

A. Viscosity.

Q 386

The Bernoulli effect describes:

a. decreased resistance distal to a stenosis

b. decreased flow volume in critical stenosis

c. decreased velocities in regions of flow turbulence

d. decreased pressure in regions of high flow speed

DAVIES Registry Reviews & Study Aids

A 386

D. Decreased pressure in regions of high flow speed.

Q 387

Why do collateral vessels tend to have higher resistance than normal flow channels?

a. small lumen diameter

b. greater length

c. higher viscosity

d. a and b

A 387

D. A and B.

Q 388

The effect of massage or pressure on the carotid sinus is to:

a. increase blood pressure

b. produce reflex bradycardia

c. increase stroke volume

d. produce tachycardia

DAVIES
Registry Reviews & Study Aids

A 388

B. Produce reflex bradycardia.

▶ Belanger AC: *Vascular Anatomy and Physiology*. Pasadena, Davies Publishing, 1999, p 75.

Q 389

Peripheral resistance is controlled by:

a. vasoconstriction and vasodilatation of the arterioles
b. muscle contraction
c. stroke volume
d. heart rate

A 389

A. Vasoconstriction and vasodilatation of the arterioles.

Q 390

The energy of something in motion is known as:

a. kinetic energy
b. potential energy
c. fluid energy
d. viscous energy

A 390

A. Kinetic energy.

Q 391

What changes would be seen in a Doppler waveform of the femoral artery that is taken after exercise?

a. no changes

b. increased reverse component in early diastole

c. delayed systolic rise time

d. increased flow throughout diastole

A 391

D. Increased flow throughout diastole.

During exercise, the muscles have greater demand for oxygenated blood. The arterioles dilate and resistance to flow decreases. As flow resistance diminishes, the volume of diastolic flow increases.

▸ Belanger AC: *Vascular Anatomy and Physiology*. Pasadena, Davies Publishing, 1999, pp 163–165.

Q 392

The Reynolds number denotes the:

a. point at which flow becomes turbulent
b. effect of arteriolar vasodilatation or vasoconstriction on flow velocity
c. point at which resistance to flow is increased in a stenosis
d. effect of pressure on volume flow

A 392

A. Point at which flow becomes turbulent.

Q 393

What factor has the greatest influence on flow resistance?

a. vessel radius

b. viscosity

c. vessel length

d. pressure gradient

A 393

A. Vessel radius.

Q 394

What does the term *laminar flow* describe?

a. the layered manner in which blood flow courses within an arterial lumen

b. turbulent flow distal to a stenosis

c. accelerated flow within a narrowed arterial segment

d. disturbed flow at arterial bifurcations

A 394

A. The layered manner in which blood flow courses within an arterial lumen.

Q 395

Which of the following accurately describes the exit effects of flow through a stenosis?

a. The flow profile elongates and eventually reestablishes as parabolic.

b. Boundary layer separation occurs.

c. Flow near the vessel edges becomes stagnant or retrograde.

d. All of the above.

DAVIES
Registry Reviews & Study Aids

A 395

D. All of the above.

Q 396

A plug flow profile would most likely be seen in which vessel?

a. external carotid artery
b. vertebral artery
c. proper hepatic artery
d. abdominal aorta

A 396

D. Abdominal aorta.

A plug or blunted flow profile is seen in large arteries such as the abdominal aorta and common carotid artery. In these arteries the central portion of the fluid moves together and a velocity gradient occurs near the wall.

▸ Belanger AC: *Vascular Anatomy and Physiology*. Pasadena, Davies Publishing, 1999, pp 123–125.

Q 397

Where in this illustration would pressure be greatest?

a. A

b. B

c. C

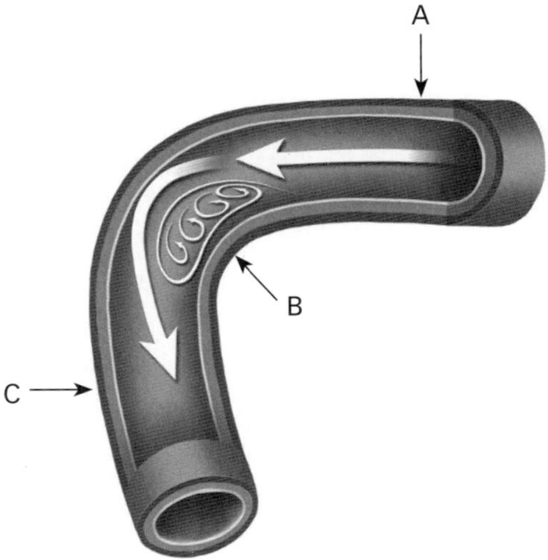

Physiology and Fluid Dynamics / Arterial Hemodynamics / AIT—Hotspot

A 397

B. B.

- Rumwell C, McPharlin M: *Vascular Technology: An Illustrated Review*, 5th edition. Pasadena, Davies Publishing, 2015, p 26.

Q 398

Where in this illustration is the location of flow separation?

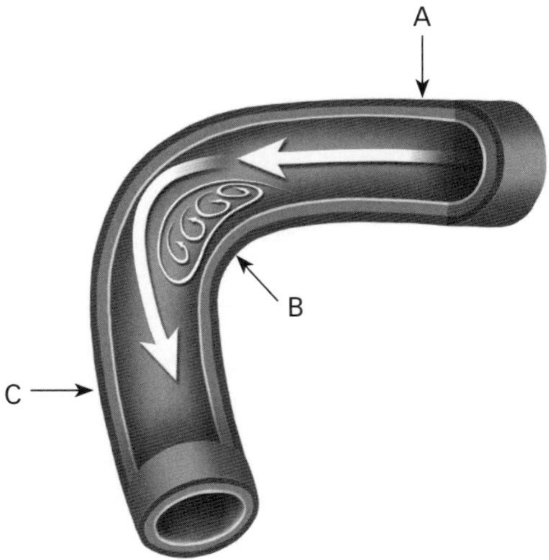

a. A

b. B

c. C

A 398

B. B.

▶ Rumwell C, McPharlin M: *Vascular Technology: An Illustrated Review*, 5th edition. Pasadena, Davies Publishing, 2015, p 26.

Q 399

Characterize velocity at point B.

a. high

b. low

c. nonexistent

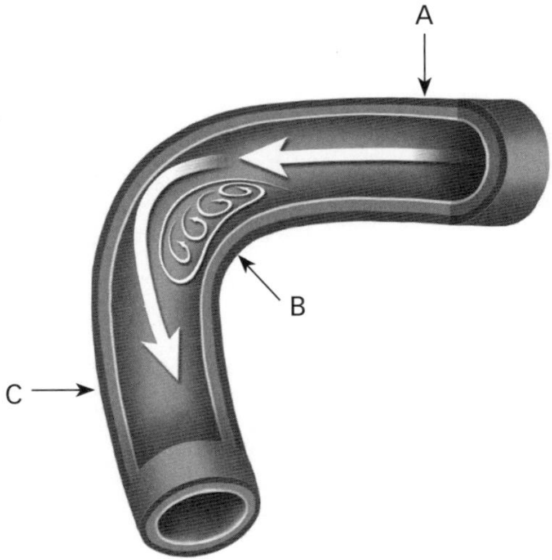

A 399

B. Low.

Pressure energy is higher and velocity energy is lower in an area of flow separation.

▶ Rumwell C, McPharlin M: *Vascular Technology: An Illustrated Review*, 5th edition. Pasadena, Davies Publishing, 2015, p 26.

Q 400

What does the term *phasicity*, in reference to the venous system, denote?

a. the ebb and flow in the veins that occurs in response to respiration

b. the rate at which the valves open and close

c. the effect of intrinsic and extrinsic pressure on venous wall stiffness

d. the influence of the cardiac cycle on venous flow

A 400

A. The ebb and flow in the veins that occurs in response to respiration.

- Rumwell C, McPharlin M: *Vascular Technology: An Illustrated Review*, 5th edition. Pasadena, Davies Publishing, 2015, pp 304–305.

Q 401

Which position would result in the greatest hydrostatic pressure?

a. Trendelenburg
b. standing
c. supine
d. Hydrostatic pressure does not vary with position.

A 401

B. Standing.

Hydrostatic pressure varies with position. It is the pressure exerted by fluid within a closed system, such as oil in a pipeline or blood in the circulatory system. Hydrostatic pressure is greatest in a standing position. In a supine position there is virtually no hydrostatic pressure.

- Rumwell C, McPharlin M: *Vascular Technology: An Illustrated Review*, 5th edition. Pasadena, Davies Publishing, 2015, pp 18–19.
- Belanger AC: *Vascular Anatomy and Physiology*. Pasadena, Davies Publishing, 1999, pp 131, 173–175.

Q 402

What is the effect of inspiration on venous flow in the lower extremities?

a. During inspiration the flow courses from the perforating veins into the superficial veins.

b. With competent valves, venous flow augments during inspiration and reverses during expiration.

c. If the calf muscle is contracted, the flow will course toward the ankle during inspiration.

d. In the supine position, venous flow in the lower extremities stops during inspiration and returns during expiration.

DAVIES Registry Reviews & Study Aids

A 402

D. In the supine position, venous flow in the lower extremities stops during inspiration and returns during expiration.

▶ Rumwell C, McPharlin M: *Vascular Technology: An Illustrated Review*, 5th edition. Pasadena, Davies Publishing, 2015, p 280.

Q 403

At any moment, how much of the body's blood volume is found in the veins?

a. 10%–20%

b. 25%–40%

c. 40%–50%

d. 60%–75%

A 403

D. 60%–75%.

▸ Belanger AC: *Vascular Anatomy and Physiology*. Pasadena, Davies Publishing, 1999, p 167.

Q 404

Which of the following would **NOT** be true regarding the lower extremity veins in an individual who has been standing for a long time?

a. Hypotension could occur due to diminished cardiac output.
b. Hydrostatic pressure would be high in the lower extremity veins.
c. Pooling of blood would occur in the lower extremity veins.
d. The veins of the lower extremity would collapse under the increased pressure.

DAVIES Registry Reviews & Study Aids

A 404

D. This statement–"the veins of the lower extremity would collapse under the increased pressure"–is **NOT** true.

In fact the veins of the lower extremity would become distended as a result of venous pooling and high pressure.

▸ Belanger AC: *Vascular Anatomy and Physiology*. Pasadena, Davies Publishing, 1999, pp 167–183.

Q 405

All of the following statements apply to the calf-muscle pump **EXCEPT**:

a. Muscular contraction increases venous return and therefore cardiac output.

b. Contraction of the muscle propels blood toward the heart.

c. Hydrostatic pressure is increased in the veins at the ankle with contraction of the muscle pump.

d. Competent valves stop blood from flowing retrograde during muscle contraction.

DAVIES
Registry Reviews & Study Aids

A 405

C. This statement–"hydrostatic pressure is increased in the veins at the ankle with contraction of the muscle pump"–is **NOT** true.

With contraction of the calf-muscle pump, the hydrostatic fluid column is interrupted and pressure is decreased in the veins at the ankle.

▶ Belanger AC: *Vascular Anatomy and Physiology*. Pasadena, Davies Publishing, 1999, pp 167–183.

Q 406

Which statement regarding intrathoracic pressure is **NOT** true?

a. Venous return from the upper extremities is reduced when intrathoracic pressure is high.

b. Intrathoracic pressure is increased with inspiration.

c. Intrathoracic pressure is increased with the Valsalva maneuver.

d. Intrathoracic pressure has a major effect on venous return.

DAVIES
Registry Reviews & Study Aids

A 406

B. This statement—"intrathoracic pressure is increased with inspiration"—is **NOT** true.

With inspiration, intrathoracic pressure decreases and intra-abdominal pressure increases. This increases venous return from the upper extremity and stops venous flow in the lower extremity. The Valsalva maneuver increases both intrathoracic and intra-abdominal pressure, which decreases venous return to the heart.

▸ Rumwell C, McPharlin M: *Vascular Technology: An Illustrated Review*, 5th edition. Pasadena, Davies Publishing, 2015, p 280.

Q 407

What is the main power source for blood propulsion in the venous system?

a. bicuspid valves

b. right atrium

c. respiration

d. calf muscle

A 407

D. Calf muscle.

Q 408

A condition in which the body tissue contains excessive fluid is termed:

a. pigmentation
b. cellulitis
c. edema
d. lymphangitis

DAVIES
Registry Reviews & Study Aids

A 408

C. Edema.

Q 409

Which of the following does **NOT** accurately describe events during calf-muscle contraction and relaxation?

a. Blood flows from the deep system into the superficial system via the perforators during relaxation.
b. A potential "space" is created with very low pressure during relaxation.
c. Blood is forced cephalad during contraction.
d. Soleal sinuses empty during contraction.

A 409

A. This statement—"blood flows from the deep system into the superficial system via the perforators during relaxation"—is **NOT** correct.

During relaxation, blood flows from the superficial system into the deep system.

▶ Rumwell C, McPharlin M: *Vascular Technology: An Illustrated Review*, 5th edition. Pasadena, Davies Publishing, 2015, p 279.

Q 410

Which of the following causes the veins to lose their elliptical shape and become more circular?

a. increased interstitial pressure

b. increased transmural pressure

c. decreased intraluminal pressure

d. decreased hydrostatic pressure

A 410

B. Increased transmural pressure.

Q 411

The type of pressure that is greatly influenced by gravity is:

a. transmural pressure
b. interstitial pressure
c. hydrostatic pressure
d. intraluminal pressure

A 411

C. Hydrostatic pressure.

Q 412

Intra-abdominal pressure is decreased with:

a. inspiration
b. Valsalva maneuver
c. a and b
d. expiration

A 412

D. Expiration.

Q 413

What is the term for the ability of veins to accommodate large shifts in volume with only limited changes in venous pressure?

a. transluminal pressure

b. augmentation

c. phasicity

d. compliance

A 413

D. Compliance.

▶ Rumwell C, McPharlin M: *Vascular Technology: An Illustrated Review*, 5th edition. Pasadena, Davies Publishing, 2015, pp 277–280.

Q 414

All of the changes below can be attributed to incompetent venous valves following venous thrombosis **EXCEPT**:

a. edema

b. varicose superficial veins

c. venous hypertension

d. venous malformation

A 414

D. Venous malformation is **NOT** attributable to incompetent venous valves.

With incompetent valves, the hydrostatic pressure column is uninterrupted from the right atrium to the lower legs. This pressure leads to venous distention and more incompetent veins in superficial veins and perforators. Secondary varicose veins develop. Edema, cellulitis, brown discoloration of the skin, and ulceration eventually may develop.

▶ Rumwell C, McPharlin M: *Vascular Technology: An Illustrated Review*, 5th edition. Pasadena, Davies Publishing, 2015, pp 278–280.

Q 415

All of the statements below are accurate regarding an arteriovenous fistula **EXCEPT**:

a. There is an increase in the volume of blood flow in the feeding artery.

b. Arterial resistance proximal to the fistula is decreased.

c. Venous pressure in draining veins is decreased.

d. High-output cardiac failure is common in large arteriovenous fistulae.

A 415

C. This statement–"venous pressure in draining veins is decreased"–is incorrect regarding an arteriovenous fistula.

Q 416

What Doppler findings would **NOT** be evident in an acute traumatic arteriovenous fistula?

a. increased diastolic flow in the feeding artery
b. prominent collateral veins around the fistula
c. pulsatile flow in the draining vein
d. increased systolic velocity in the feeding artery

DAVIES
Registry Reviews & Study Aids

A 416

B. Prominent collateral veins around the fistula would **NOT** be evident in this situation.

In an acute setting, collateral vessels have not had time to develop. All other statements are true.

Q 417

Which statement is **NOT** true regarding arteriovenous malformations?

a. They can be defined as a direct connection between an artery and a vein.
b. They are present at birth.
c. They may be asymptomatic.
d. They can occur anywhere in the body.

DAVIES
Registry Reviews & Study Aids

A 417

A. This statement–"they can be defined as a direct connection between an artery and a vein"–is **NOT** true.

An arteriovenous *fistula* is a direct communication between an artery and a vein. An arteriovenous *malformation* is present at birth and is an abnormal network in which arterial afferents flow directly into venous efferents without an intervening capillary bed.

Q 418

Which of the following complications can occur with hemodialysis access grafts?

a. pseudoaneurysm

b. distal limb ischemia

c. congestive heart failure

d. all of the above

DAVIES
Registry Reviews & Study Aids

A 418

D. All of the above.

Q 419

Trauma can result in all of the following **EXCEPT**:

a. arteriovenous malformation

b. pseudoaneurysm

c. arteriovenous fistula

d. dissection

A 419

A. Arteriovenous malformation.

Arteriovenous fistulae, pseudoaneurysms, and dissections commonly occur as a result of trauma. An arteriovenous malformation may be exacerbated by trauma but is present at birth.

Q 420

In this image from a 48-year-old male, a large paraumbilical vein is seen exiting the liver. This is indicative of:

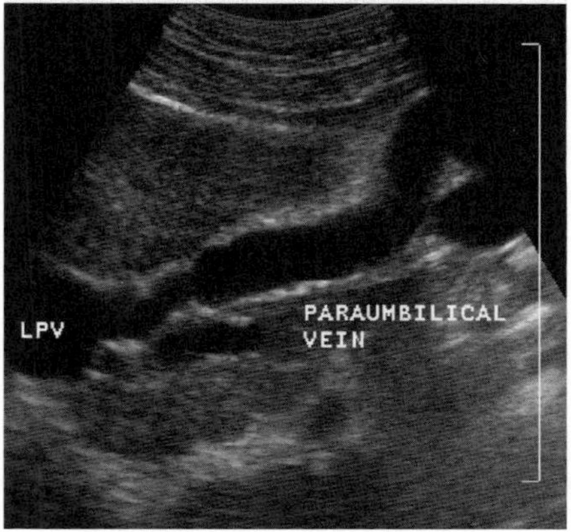

a. arteriovenous fistula between the hepatic and portal venous systems
b. main portal vein thrombosis
c. portal hypertension
d. hepatofugal flow in the main portal vein

A 420

C. Portal hypertension.

Although not all patients with portal hypertension develop an enlarged paraumbilical vein, its presence is diagnostic of the disorder. The paraumbilical vein is a vestige of the umbilical circulation in the fetus. The paraumbilical vein(s) connect the portal venous system to the systemic venous system, forming a portosystemic shunt.

Q 421

This image is from a 64-year-old male with back pain. Which term best describes the aortic aneurysm?

a. ectatic

b. saccular

c. mycotic

d. fusiform

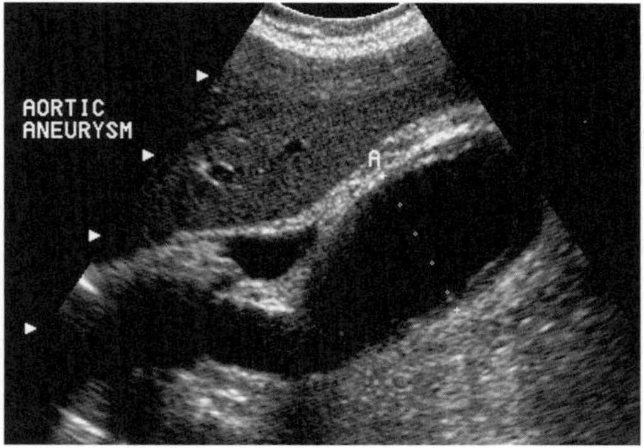

A 421

D. Fusiform.

A fusiform aneurysm is a circumferential enlargement of a segment of the artery and is the most common aneurysm shape. A saccular aneurysm is a focal outpouching of an artery. A mycotic aneurysm is one that has become infected; the term *mycotic* does not describe a specific aneurysmal shape. An ectatic artery is one that is dilated but not aneurysmal by definition.

▶ Rumwell C, McPharlin M: *Vascular Technology: An Illustrated Review*, 5th edition. Pasadena, Davies Publishing, 2015, pp 48–49.

Q 422

How would this angiogram be interpreted?

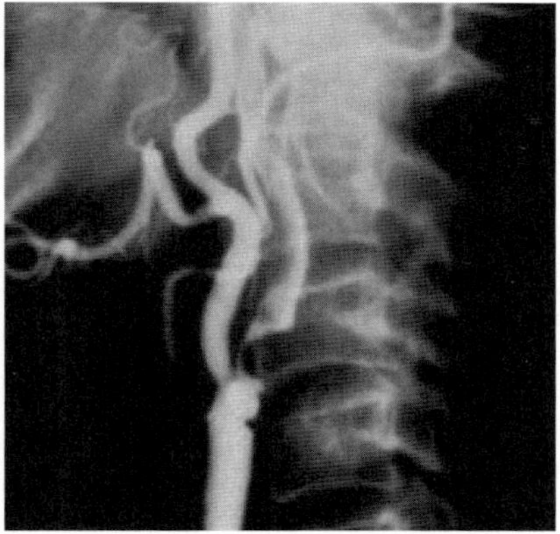

a. This patient has a hemodynamically significant lesion of the external carotid artery.

b. This film documents a preocclusive lesion of the internal carotid artery.

c. This study shows a severe problem with the distal common carotid artery.

d. You suspect an occluded internal carotid artery.

A 422

B. This film documents a preocclusive lesion of the internal carotid artery.

▶ Rumwell C, McPharlin M: *Vascular Technology: An Illustrated Review*, 5th edition. Pasadena, Davies Publishing, 2015, pp 389, 404.

Q 423

This image of the common carotid artery is from a 36-year-old female with Marfan syndrome. The linear structure indicated by the arrow represents an intimal flap. Which of the following conditions is present?

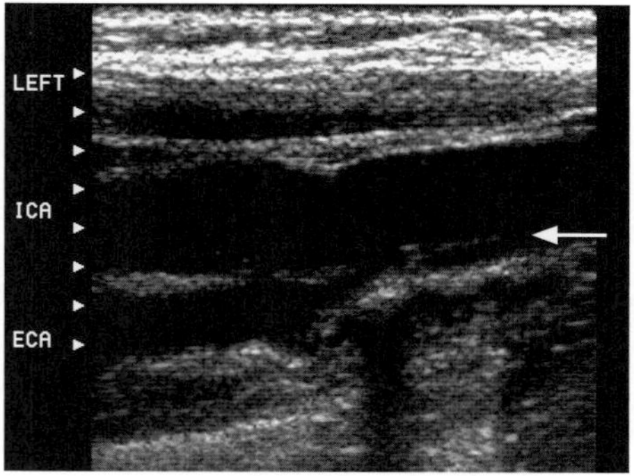

a. arterial dissection

b. pseudoaneurysm

c. fibromuscular hyperplasia

d. arteriovenous fistula

A 423

A. Arterial dissection.

Q 424

This image of the popliteal vein is from a 46-year-old female with leg swelling. Which of the following correctly describes the ultrasound findings?

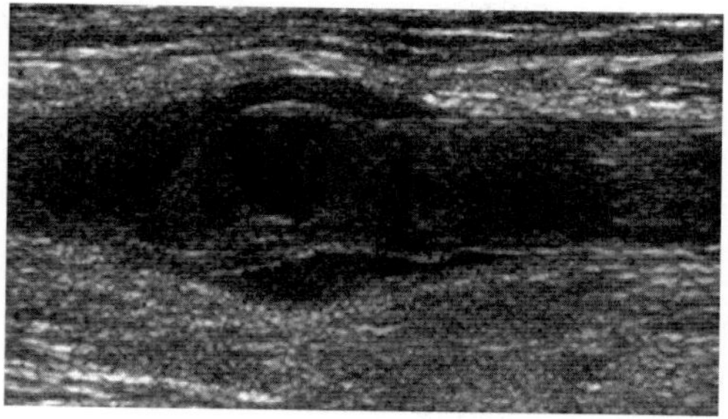

a. Baker's cyst

b. chronic thrombus in the popliteal vein

c. acute thrombus in the popliteal vein

d. rouleau formation in the popliteal vein

A 424

C. Acute thrombus in the popliteal vein.

Q 425

This waveform profile is characteristic of which of the following?

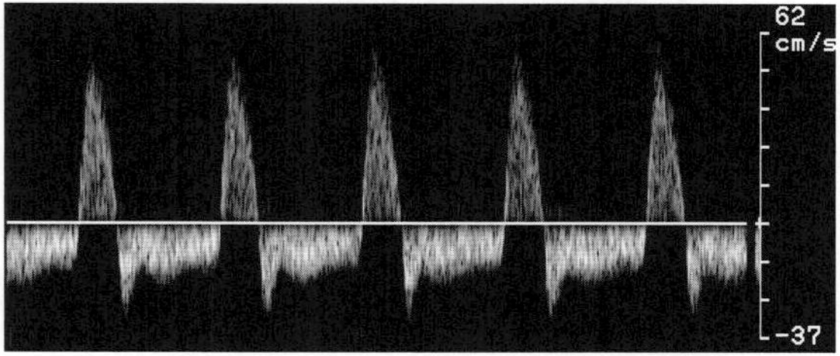

a. neck of pseudoaneurysm

b. arteriovenous communication

c. dampened signal obtained proximal to arterial occlusion

d. hyperemic flow

A 425

A. Neck of pseudoaneurysm.

Q 426

Which term can be used to describe this waveform?

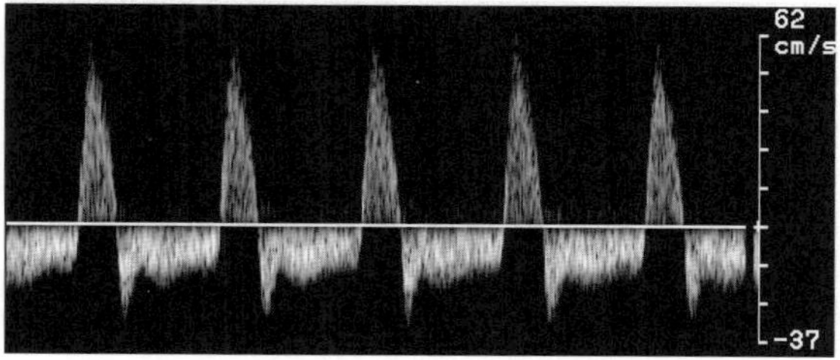

a. monophasic
b. hepatofugal
c. bidirectional
d. tardus parvus

A 426

C. Bidirectional.

Q 427

This waveform profile is characteristic of which of the following?

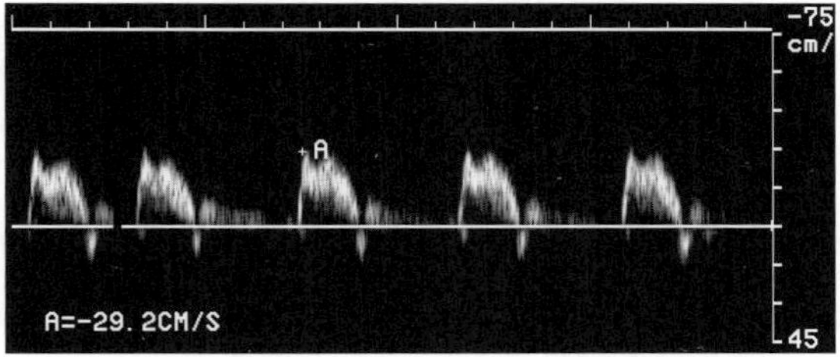

a. neck of pseudoaneurysm

b. dampened signal obtained proximal to arterial occlusion

c. arteriovenous communication

d. hyperemic flow

DAVIES
Registry Reviews & Study Aids

A 427

B. Dampened signal obtained proximal to arterial occlusion.

Q 428

Which term can be used to describe this waveform?

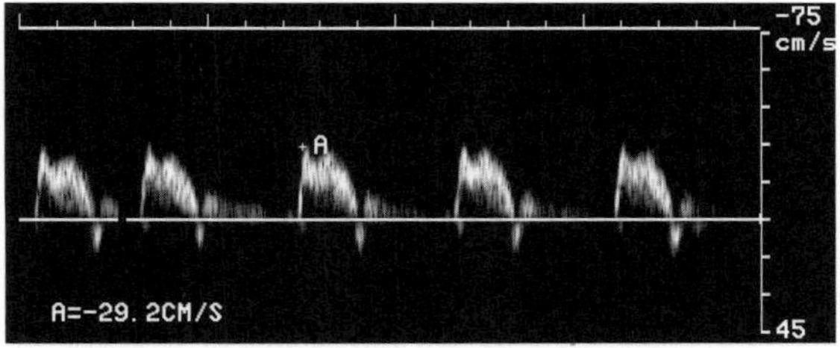

a. triphasic

b. biphasic

c. tardus parvus

d. monophasic

A 428

A. Triphasic.

Q 429

The end-diastolic portion of this external carotid artery waveform is not demonstrated on this image because:

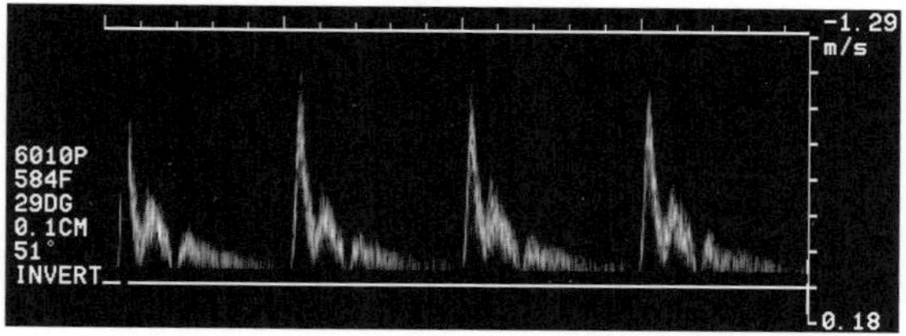

a. the Doppler frequency is too high

b. the pulse repetition frequency is set too low

c. the Doppler angle is too great

d. the wall filter is set too high

A 429

D. The wall filter is set too high.

Q 430

Which statement is **TRUE** regarding measurements obtained from this waveform?

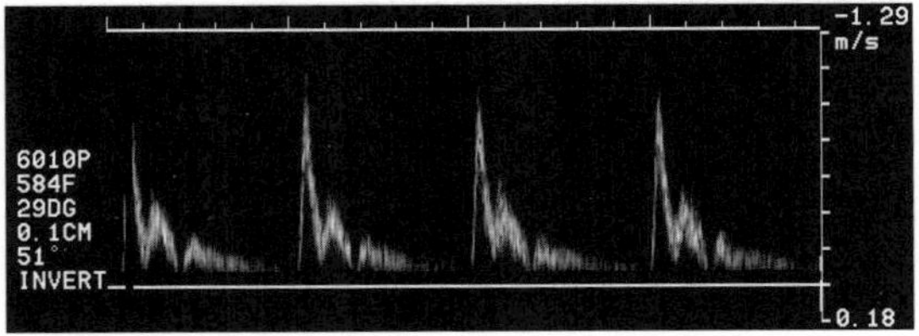

a. The pulsatility index would be erroneously low.

b. The acceleration time would be erroneously short.

c. The resistive index would be erroneously high.

d. The peak systolic velocity would be erroneously low.

DAVIES
Registry Reviews & Study Aids

A 430

C. The resistive index would be erroneously high.

Q 431

This waveform was obtained at the porta hepatis in a patient with portal hypertension. The signals from both the portal vein and the hepatic artery are demonstrated. Which of the following statements is correct?

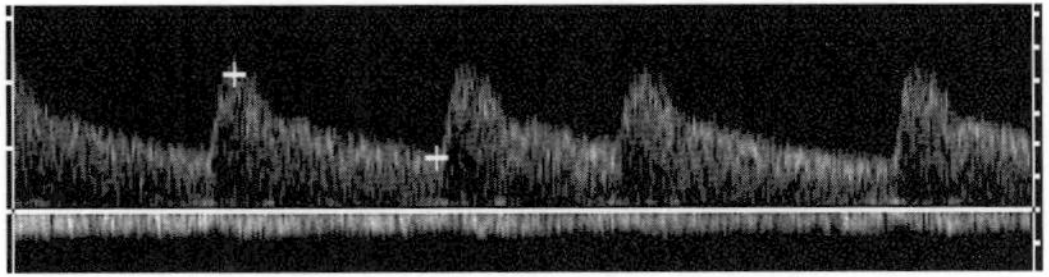

a. Hepatofugal flow is present in the portal vein.

b. Hepatofugal flow is present in the hepatic artery.

c. The hepatic artery shows a high-resistance waveform pattern.

d. A fistula is present between the portal vein and hepatic artery.

A 431

A. Hepatofugal flow is present in the portal vein.

Q 432

What clinical condition is associated with the findings seen in this waveform?

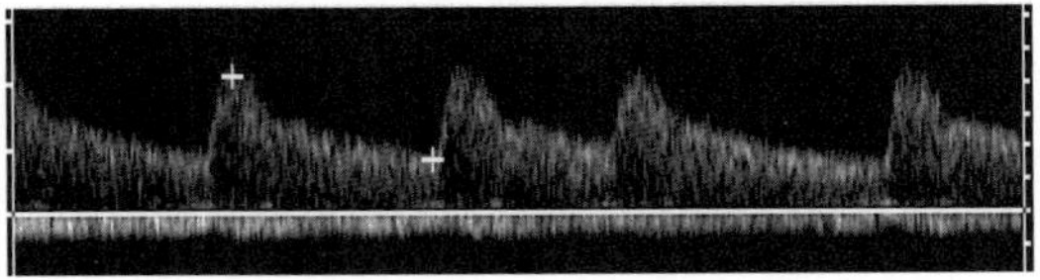

a. hepatic rejection

b. portal hypertension

c. hepatitis

d. right heart failure

A 432

B. Portal hypertension.

Q 433

This waveform was obtained in the internal carotid artery. What technical problem is present?

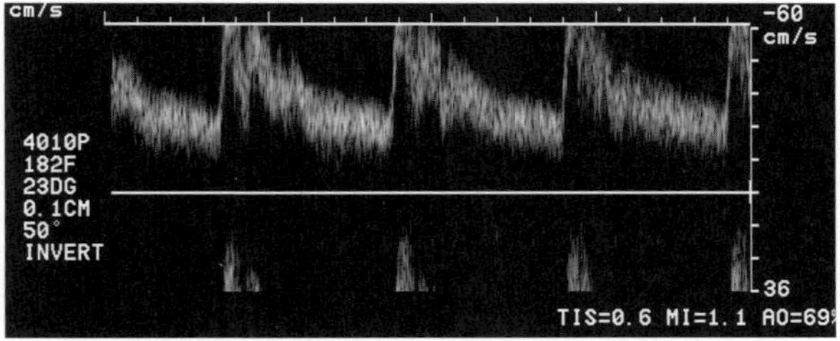

a. The baseline is set too low.

b. Aliasing is present.

c. The wall filter is set too high.

d. The pulse repetition frequency is too high.

A 433

B. Aliasing is present.

Q 434

The technical problem demonstrated in this waveform could result in which of the following errors?

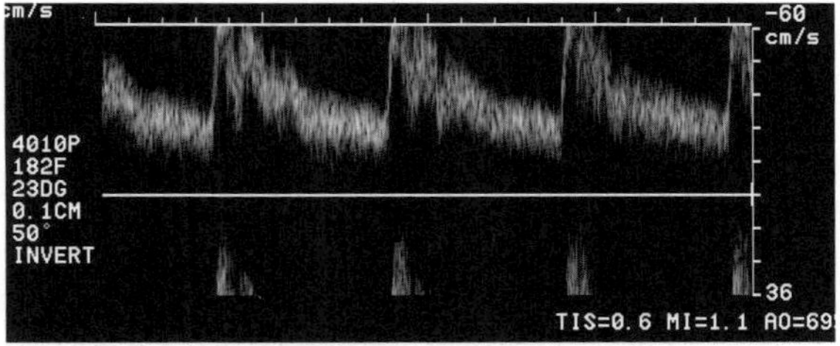

a. underestimation of end-diastolic velocity

b. overestimation of acceleration time

c. underestimation of peak systolic velocity

d. overestimation of the resistive index

DAVIES Registry Reviews & Study Aids

A 434

C. Underestimation of peak systolic velocity.

Q 435

Which of the following would **NOT** correct the technical problem demonstrated in this waveform?

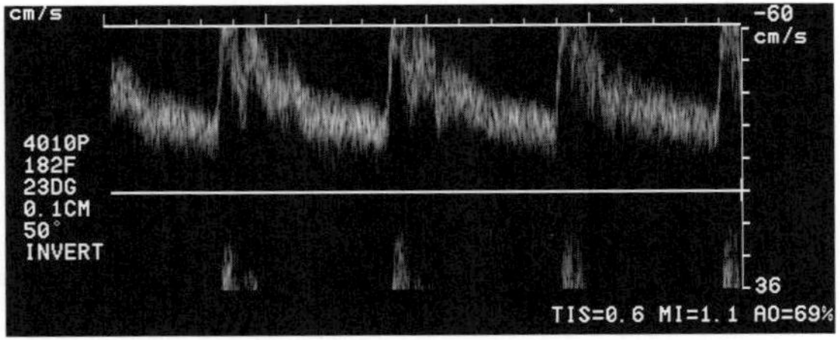

a. lower the zero baseline

b. increase the pulse repetition frequency

c. decrease the Doppler frequency

d. decrease the wall filter

A 435

D. Decrease the wall filter.

Q 436

This image is from a 22-year-old female with abnormal liver function tests and ascites. The thrombus in the inferior vena cava is most likely related to which of the following?

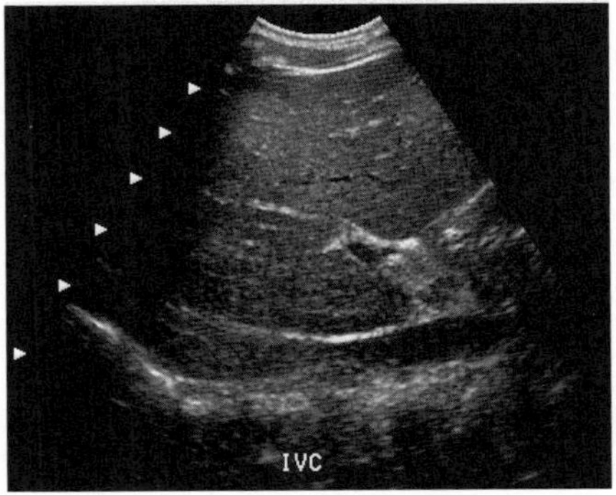

a. Takayasu's arteritis

b. Budd-Chiari syndrome

c. portal hypertension

d. cavernous transformation

A 436

B. Budd-Chiari syndrome.

Q 437

In the case described in question 436, which other abdominal vessel(s) should be evaluated for patency?

a. portal vein
b. hepatic artery
c. hepatic veins
d. a and c

A 437

D. A and C.

Q 438

Name the vessels labeled A–C:

a. ______________________________

b. ______________________________

c. ______________________________

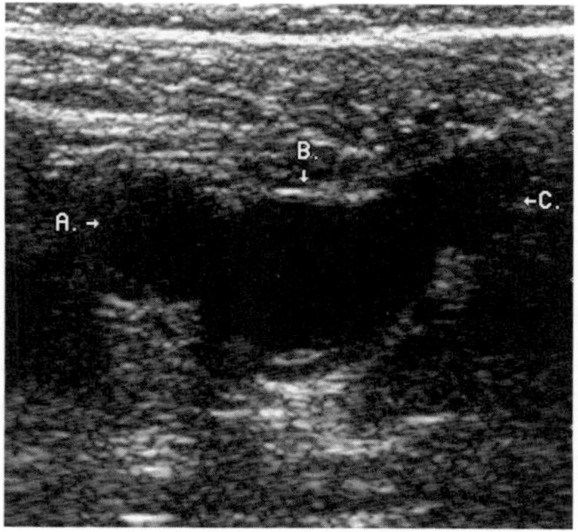

DAVIES
Registry Reviews & Study Aids

A 438

A. Common femoral artery.

B. Common femoral vein.

C. Great saphenous vein.

Q 439

This image was taken:

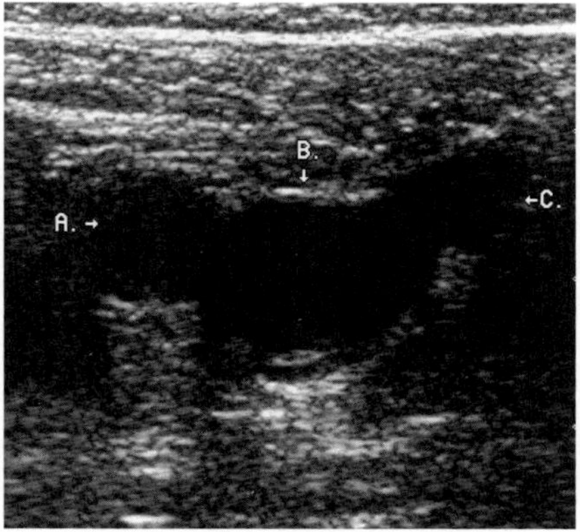

a. at the level of the inguinal ligament

b. at the level of the knee

c. at the adductor canal

d. in the neck

DAVIES
Registry Reviews & Study Aids

A 439

A. At the level of the inguinal ligament.

Q 440

Name the structures labeled A and B:

a. ______________________________

b. ______________________________

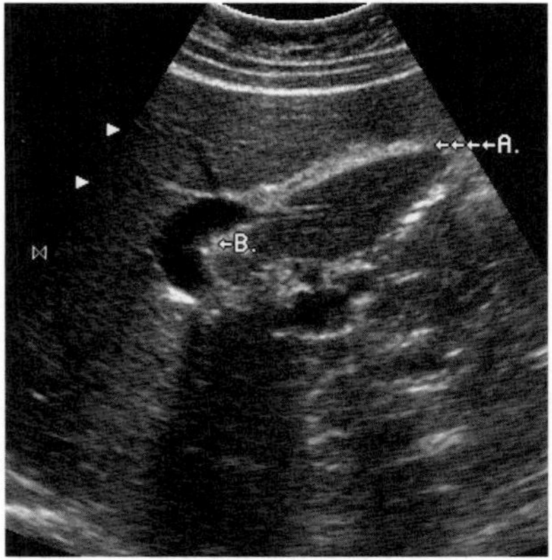

DAVIES
Registry Reviews & Study Aids

A 440

A. Ligamentum teres.

B. Left portal vein.

Q 441

Which of the following conditions is ruled out by this image?

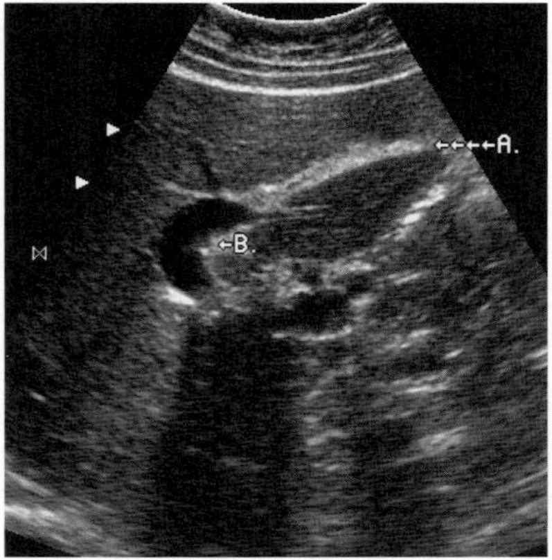

a. cavernous transformation
b. hepatic vein thrombosis
c. presence of a paraumbilical vein
d. splenic vein thrombosis

DAVIES
Registry Reviews & Study Aids

A 441

C. Presence of a paraumbilical vein.

Q 442

Name the vessels labeled A–C:

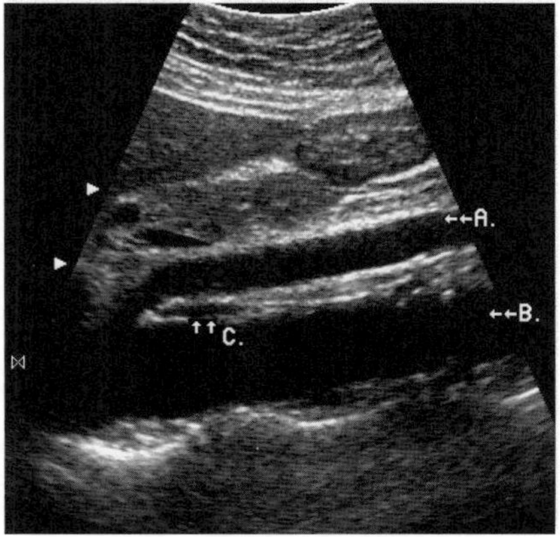

a. ______________________

b. ______________________

c. ______________________

A 442

A. Superior mesenteric artery (SMA).

B. Abdominal aorta.

C. Left renal vein (LRV).

Q 443

This image was obtained in which scan plane?

a. coronal

b. sagittal

c. oblique

d. transverse

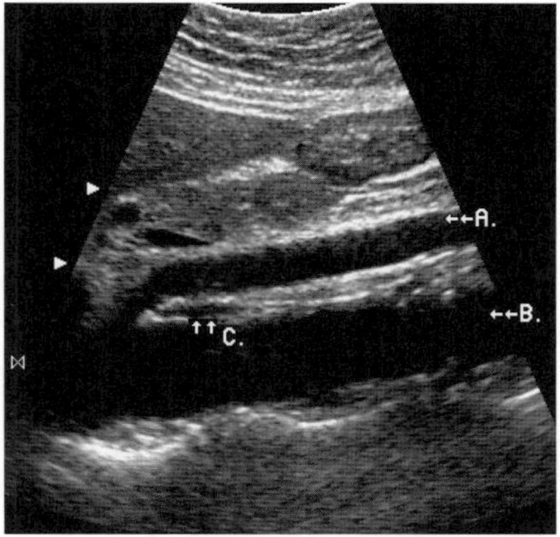

DAVIES
Registry Reviews & Study Aids

A 443

B. Sagittal.

Q 444

This image is from a 48-year-old male with increasing abdominal girth and a history of alcohol abuse. Which condition is most likely?

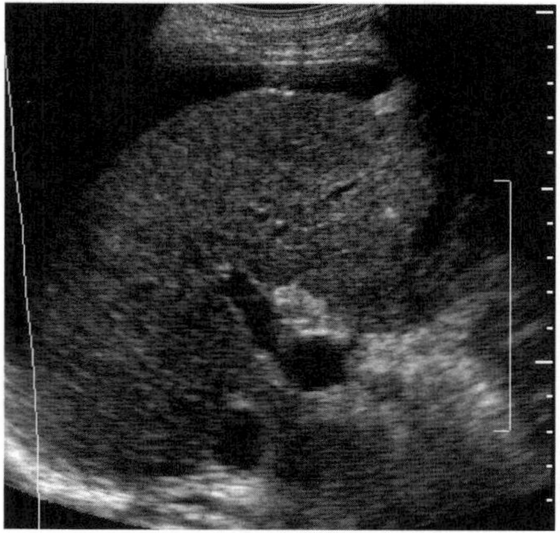

a. hepatic artery stenosis

b. portal hypertension

c. Budd-Chiari syndrome

d. cavernous transformation of the portal vein

A 444

B. Portal hypertension.

Q 445

In this B-mode image, name the vessel seen in cross section underneath the inferior vena cava.

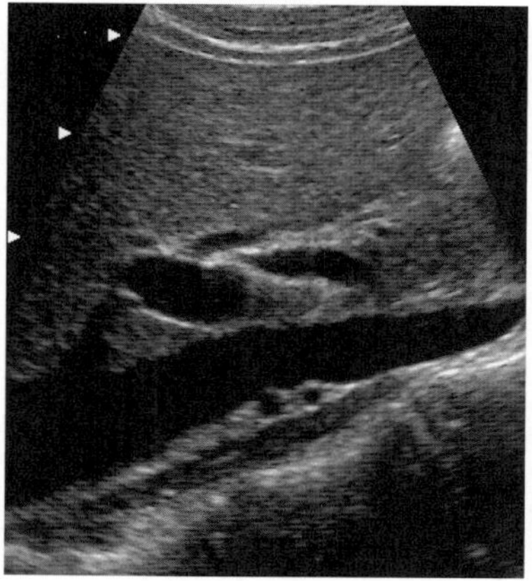

A 445

Right renal artery.

The right renal artery passes underneath the inferior vena cava as it courses to the hilum of the kidney.

Q 446

In this B-mode image, what variant vascular anatomy is present?

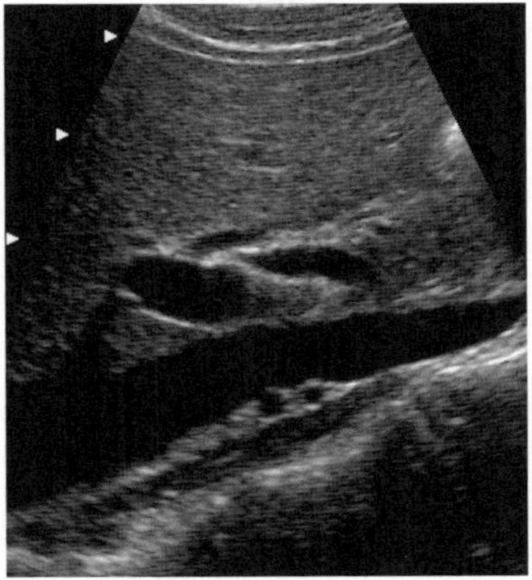

DAVIES
Registry Reviews & Study Aids

A 446

Multiple renal arteries.

There are two renal arteries in this image posterior to the inferior vena cava. Multiple renal arteries occur in up to 20% of individuals. In the evaluation of the renal arteries for stenosis in renovascular hypertension, each renal artery identified must be evaluated throughout its length. The presence of unidentified accessory or supernumerary renal arteries is a potential pitfall in the ultrasound evaluation for renal artery stenosis.

Q 447

This Doppler waveform was obtained in a stenotic femoral artery. Was it most likely taken proximal or distal to the site of stenosis?

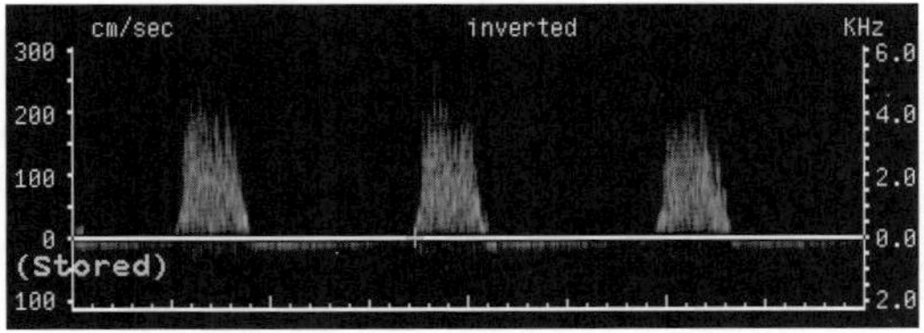

A 447

Distal.

This waveform demonstrates poststenotic turbulence. This can be seen in the fill-in of the spectral window and the presence of a small amount of flow below the zero baseline.

Q 448

Which term can be used to describe this waveform?

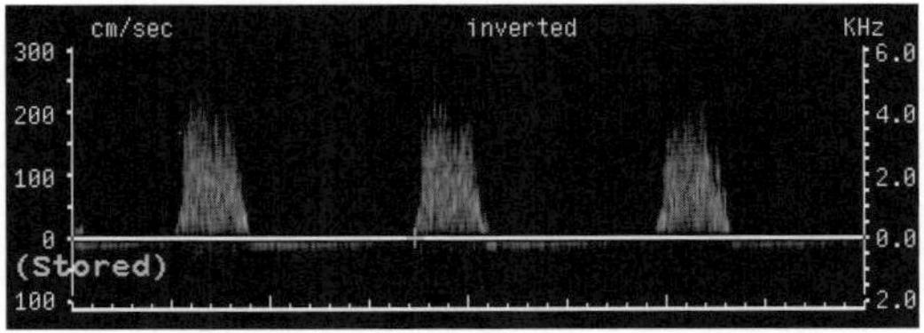

a. monophasic

b. tardus parvus

c. phasic

d. spectral broadening

DAVIES
Registry Reviews & Study Aids

A 448

D. Spectral broadening.

Q 449

What technical problem is present in this duplex sampling of the common carotid artery?

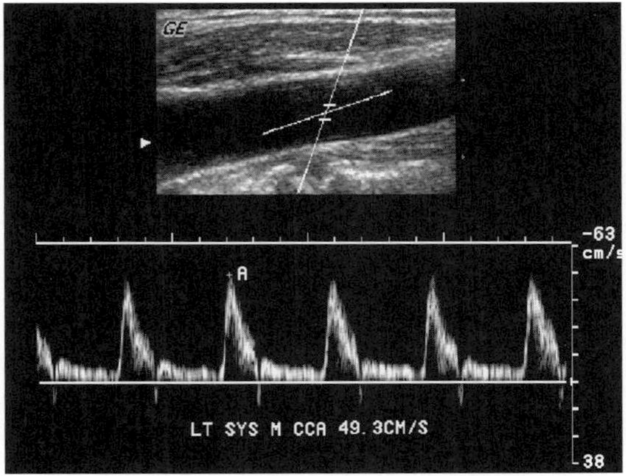

a. incorrect pulse repetition frequency

b. wall filter set incorrectly

c. incorrect measurement of the Doppler angle

d. Doppler gain too high

A 449

C. Incorrect measurement of the Doppler angle.

The Doppler angle should be aligned parallel to the vessel walls at the point of sampling.

Q 450

What error could result from the technical problem shown in question 449?

a. overestimation of peak velocity

b. erroneous display of spectral broadening

c. overestimation of systolic acceleration time

d. underestimation of peak velocity

A 450

D. Underestimation of peak velocity.

Misalignment of the Doppler angle will result in inaccurate velocity calculations. If the measured angle is smaller than the actual angle, the velocity will be underestimated. If the measured angle is larger than the actual angle, the velocity will be overestimated.

Q 451

Name the vessels labeled A–D.

a. ______________________

b. ______________________

c. ______________________

d. ______________________

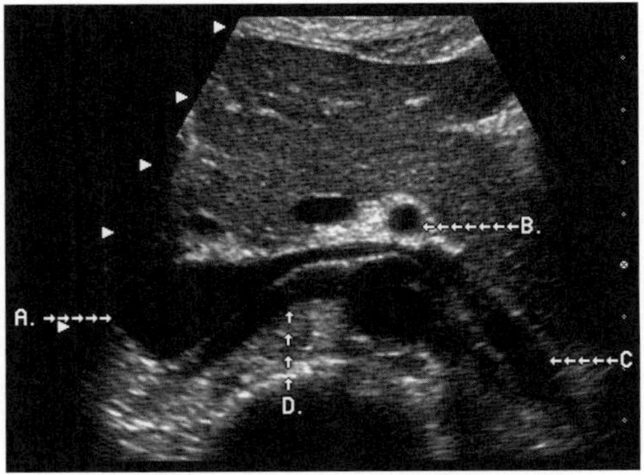

A 451

A. IVC.

B. SMA.

C. Left renal vein.

D. Right renal artery.

Q 452

This sagittal abdominal image shows a Greenfield filter positioned within which vessel?

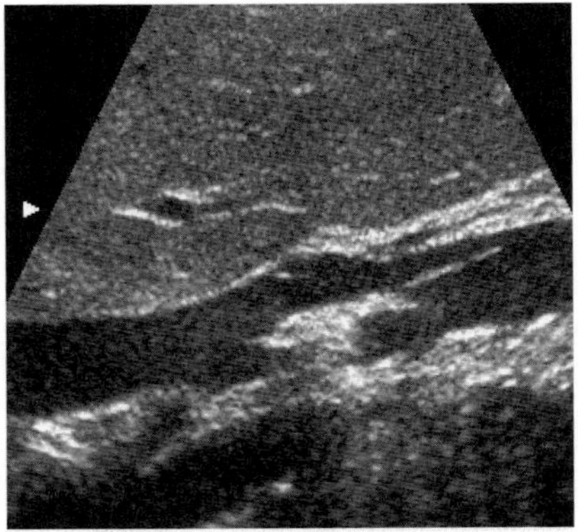

a. portal vein

b. inferior vena cava

c. abdominal aorta

d. hepatic vein

DAVIES
Registry Reviews & Study Aids

A 452

B. Inferior vena cava.

Q 453

Name the anatomy demonstrated adjacent to the aorta in this transverse image of an abdominal aortic aneurysm.

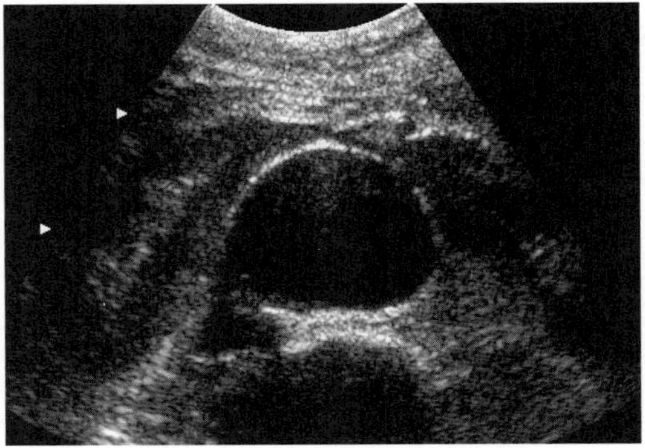

a. lymphadenopathy

b. retroperitoneal fibrosis

c. horseshoe kidneys

d. hematoma

A 453

C. Horseshoe kidneys.

Horseshoe kidneys are an anatomic variant in which both kidneys are connected at their lower (or, rarely, upper) poles across the midline. This can be a complicating factor in aortic surgery.

Q 454

What term can be used to describe the atherosclerotic plaque in this sagittal image of the internal carotid artery?

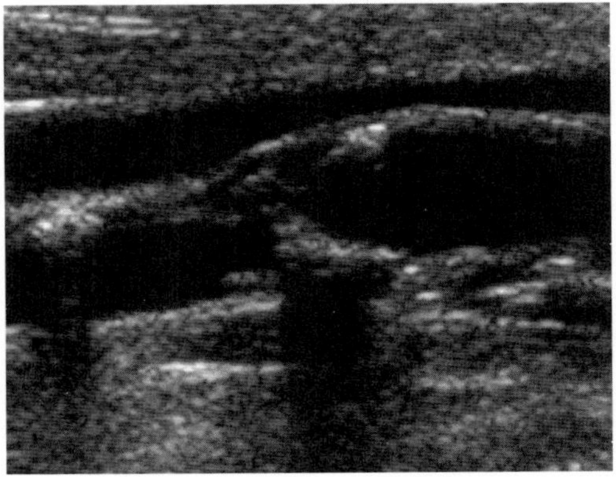

a. homogeneous

b. heterogeneous

c. smooth

d. a and c

DAVIES
Registry Reviews & Study Aids

A 454

B. Heterogeneous.

Q 455

This waveform was most likely obtained from which abdominal vessel?

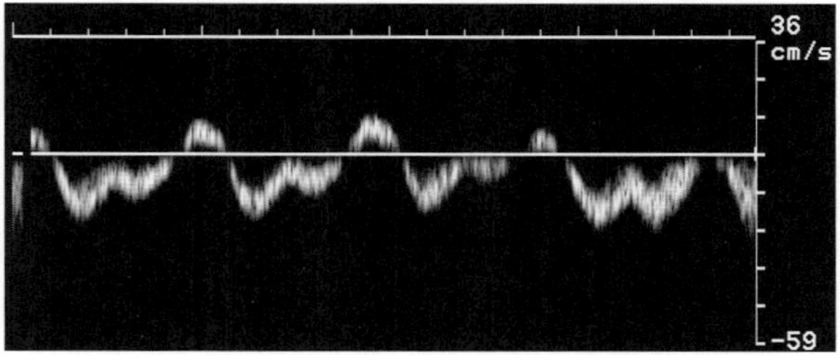

a. portal vein

b. superior mesenteric vein

c. splenic vein

d. hepatic vein

A 455

D. Hepatic vein.

Q 456

This image was obtained just below the inguinal ligament in a 37-year-old female with leg swelling. Which of the following accurately describes the ultrasound findings?

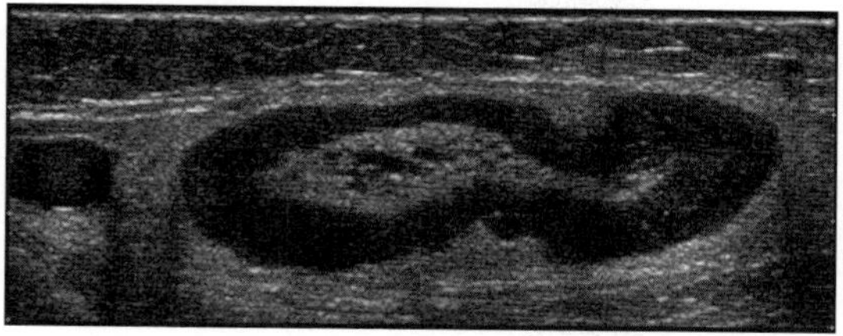

a. reactive lymph nodes

b. acute DVT of the common femoral vein

c. thigh sarcoma

d. Baker's cyst

A 456

A. Reactive lymph nodes.

Q 457

This waveform was obtained from which abdominal vessel?

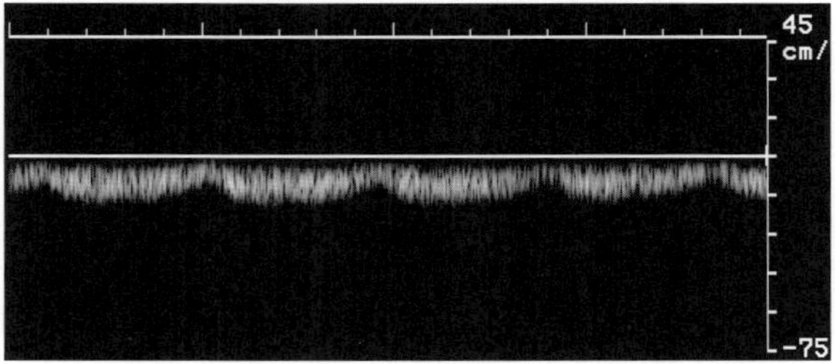

a. inferior vena cava

b. inferior mesenteric artery

c. hepatic vein

d. renal vein

A 457

D. Renal vein.

The inferior vena cava and hepatic veins demonstrate highly pulsatile waveforms. The renal vein waveform shows respiratory phasicity but minimal pulsatility.

Q 458

This sagittal image was obtained in the popliteal fossa in a patient with blue toe syndrome. What are the ultrasound findings?

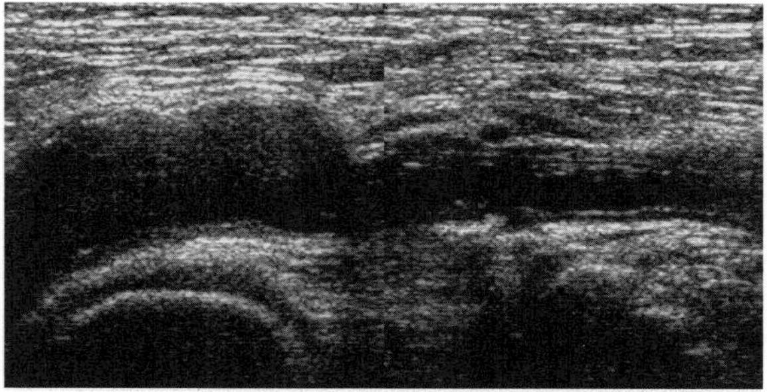

a. popliteal cyst

b. acute DVT of the popliteal vein

c. popliteal artery aneurysm

d. reactive lymph nodes

A 458

C. Popliteal artery aneurysm.

Q 459

This is a transverse image from the mid calf. Name the bones labeled A and B.

a. ______________________________

b. ______________________________

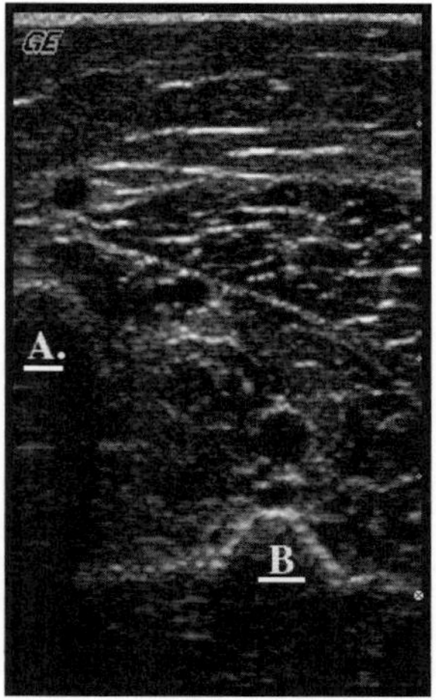

A 459

A. Tibia.

B. Fibula.

Q 460

This transverse image was obtained in the upper arm. The brachial artery is seen with a brachial vein on each side. The small arrows are pointing to what vessel?

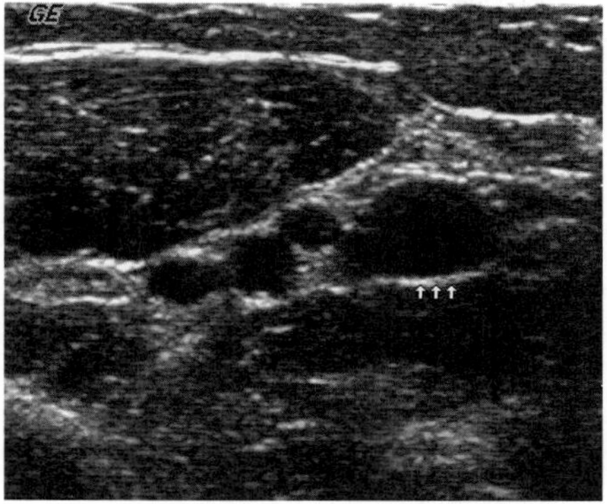

a. accessory brachial vein

b. cephalic vein

c. axillary vein

d. basilic vein

A 460

D. Basilic vein.

Q 461

This B-mode image was obtained in the upper calf. Name the vessels labeled A–F.

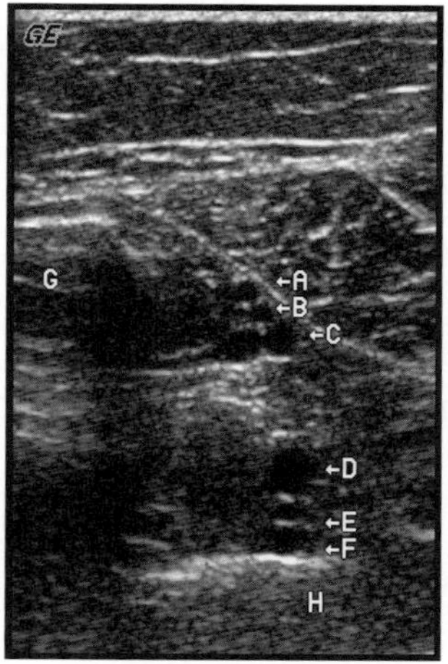

a. ______________________________

b. ______________________________

c. ______________________________

d. ______________________________

e. ______________________________

f. ______________________________

A 461

A. Posterior tibial vein.

B. Posterior tibial artery.

C. Posterior tibial vein.

D. Peroneal vein.

E. Peroneal artery.

F. Peroneal vein.

Q 462

This waveform was obtained from the left vertebral artery. From this waveform, it can be determined that there is a stenosis in what vessel?

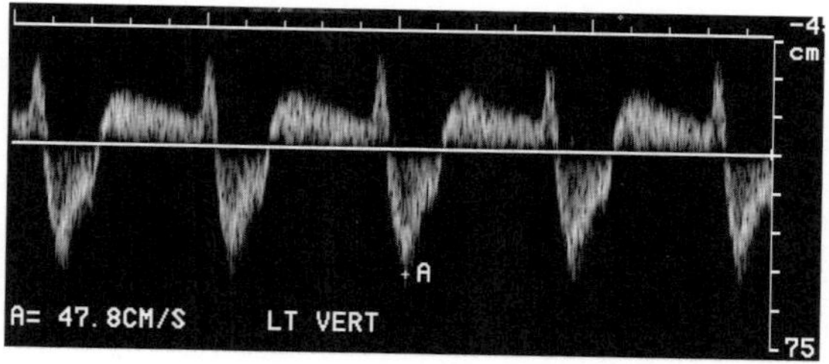

a. proximal left subclavian artery

b. innominate artery

c. distal left vertebral

d. distal left subclavian artery

A 462

A. Proximal left subclavian artery.

Q 463

This is a transverse image of the left common carotid artery. Which statement below correctly describes this image?

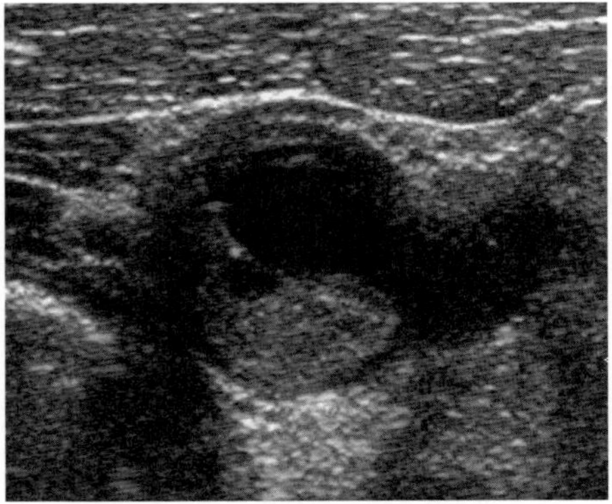

a. homogeneous plaque with calcification

b. heterogeneous plaque with questionable intraplaque hemorrhage

c. smooth homogeneous plaque

d. ulcerated plaque

A 463

B. Heterogeneous plaque with questionable intraplaque hemorrhage.

Q 464

This waveform was obtained from a fasting patient. Which vessel below is the most likely source for this Doppler trace?

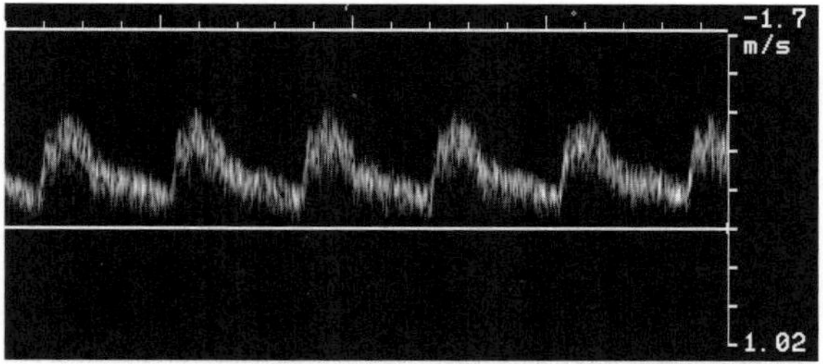

a. superior mesenteric artery

b. inferior mesenteric artery

c. infrarenal abdominal aorta

d. celiac trunk

A 464

D. Celiac trunk.

Q 465

This Doppler waveform was obtained in a posterior tibial artery by sweeping the Doppler sample volume from above (proximal to) a graft anastomosis to below (distal to) the graft anastomosis. There is retrograde flow above the bypass graft anastomotic site. What is suggested by this finding?

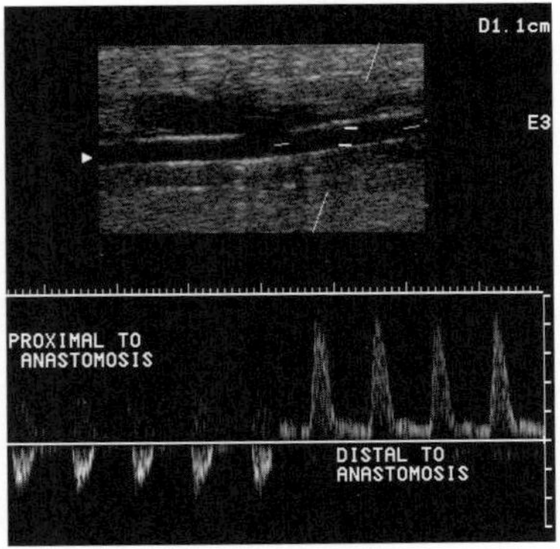

a. arteriovenous fistula proximal to the graft anastomosis
b. stenosis in the distal native artery
c. normal backflow up the native artery
d. stenosis in the graft

A 465

C. Normal backflow up the native artery.

Q 466

This Doppler waveform was obtained in a normal internal carotid artery. Which of the following could explain the loss of the spectral window?

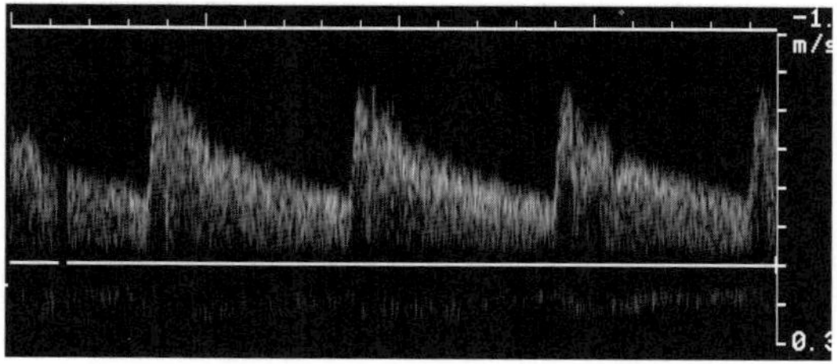

a. sweep speed set too low

b. sample volume size too small

c. pulse repetition frequency too low

d. sample volume not centered in the artery

A 466

D. Sample volume not centered in the artery.

Q 467

This sagittal image was taken from the mid calf. The vein seen in this image emptied into a posterior tibial vein. What vein is being imaged?

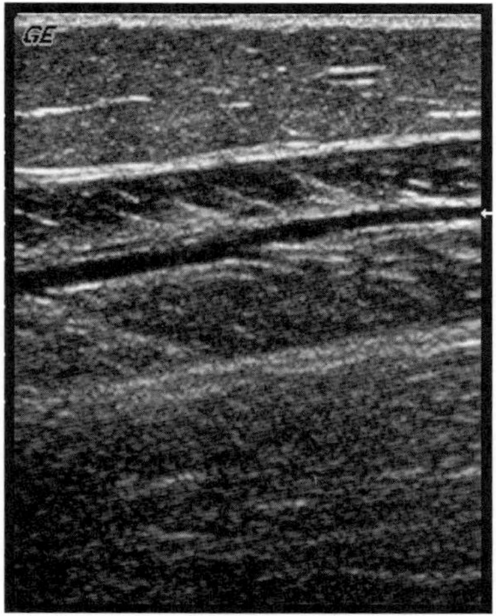

a. soleal vein

b. sural vein

c. gastrocnemius vein

d. great saphenous vein

A 467

A. Soleal vein.

Q 468

This sagittal B-mode image was taken with the probe positioned on the medial aspect of the mid calf. What pair of veins is being demonstrated?

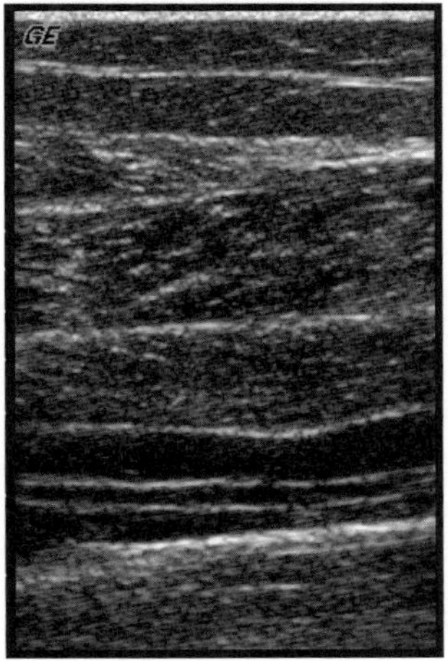

a. posterior tibial veins

b. peroneal veins

c. small saphenous veins

d. soleal veins

A 468

B. Peroneal veins.

Q 469

You acquired this image from the proximal and distal thigh of a patient a few months after fem-pop PTFE bypass graft surgery. (The echoes within the graft are from the color flow display, reproduced here in black and white.) What do you suspect?

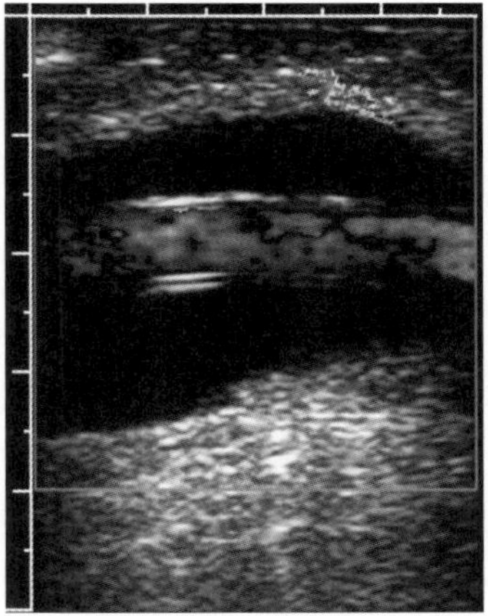

a. deep vein thrombosis

b. severe graft stenosis

c. graft occlusion

d. graft infection

A 469

D. Graft infection.

The huge area of fluid accumulation around the graft is characteristic of graft infection. Note the double-wall echo created by the graft. This appearance is characteristic of PTFE material.

Q 470

What structure in this arteriogram does the arrow point toward?

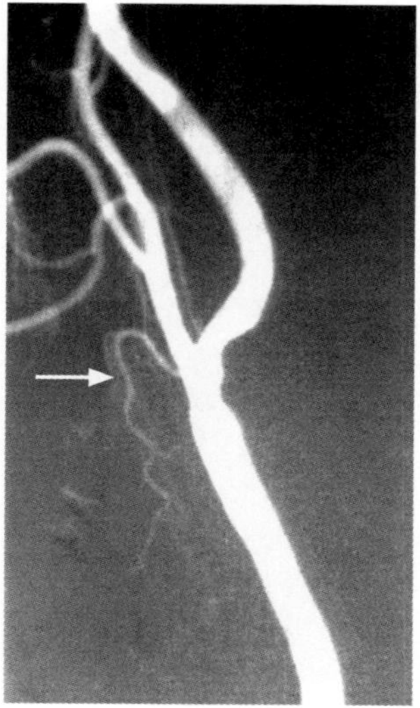

a. the superior thyroid artery

b. the facial artery

c. the angular artery

d. the superficial temporal artery

A 470

A. The superior thyroid artery.

The superior thyroid artery is the first branch of the external carotid artery, arising from the ECA near its origin and then traveling caudad.

Q 471

This angiogram of the lower extremities demonstrates:

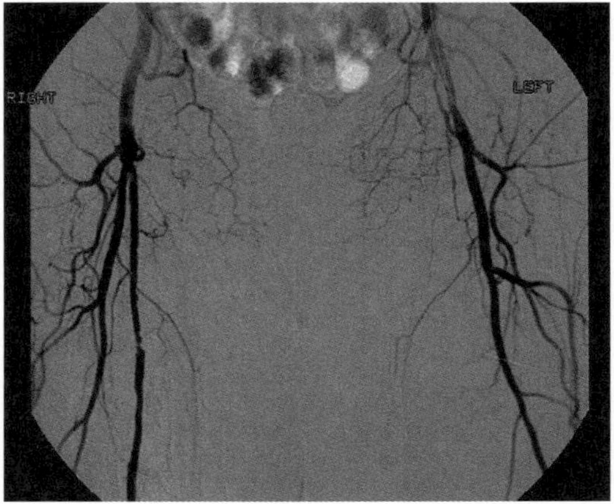

a. severe left SFA stenosis
b. severe right CFA stenosis
c. severe right SFA stenosis
d. severe left CFA stenosis

DAVIES
Registry Reviews & Study Aids

A 471

C. Severe right SFA stenosis.

There is also some diffuse irregularity along the right superficial femoral artery. A filling defect demonstrates a severe focal lesion about three-fifths of the way down this segment.

Q 472

This angiogram was taken in the AP (anteroposterior) view. What does it show?

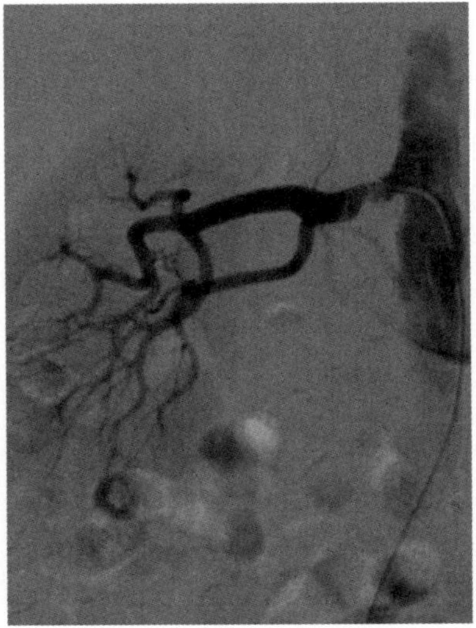

a. right renal artery stenosis
b. left renal artery stenosis
c. left renal artery occlusion
d. right renal artery occlusion

A 472

A. Right renal artery stenosis.

This is an AP view (patient's right is to your left) of a right renal artery stenosis just prior to a stenting procedure.

Q 473

The scooped-out appearance (arrow) in this image is suggestive of:

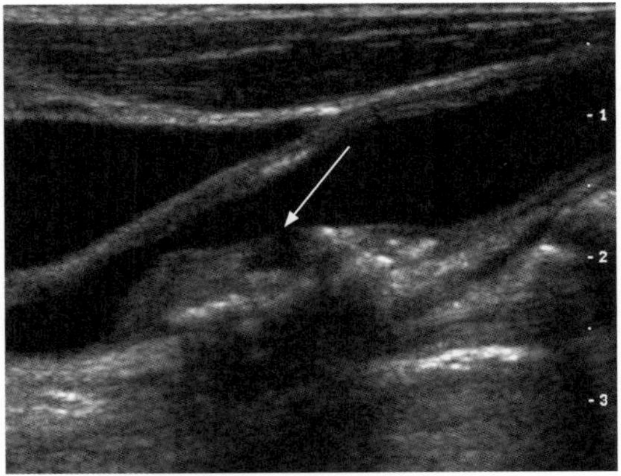

a. smooth homogeneous plaque

b. ulcerated plaque

c. homogeneous plaque with calcification

d. heterogeneous plaque with questionable intraplaque hemorrhage

DAVIES
Registry Reviews & Study Aids

A 473

B. Ulcerated plaque.

Atherosclerotic plaque causes cerebrovascular symptoms by restricting flow through hemodynamically significant lesions and by generating emboli from ulcerated plaque. The relative incidence of the two is unclear, but growing importance is being attached to the ulcerative/embolic phenomenon. Duplex scanning is quite accurate in assessing hemodynamically significant lesions, but it has been less successful in identifying ulcerative lesions that may cause embolic events. The shape that is most suggestive of ulcerated plaque is a scooped-out crater-like appearance, especially if there are shelf-like projections over the crater.

▸ Ridgway DP: *Introduction to Vascular Scanning: A Guide for the Complete Beginner*, 4th edition. Pasadena, Davies Publishing, 2014, pp 26, 77.

Q 474

What does this transverse image from the abdominal aorta demonstrate?

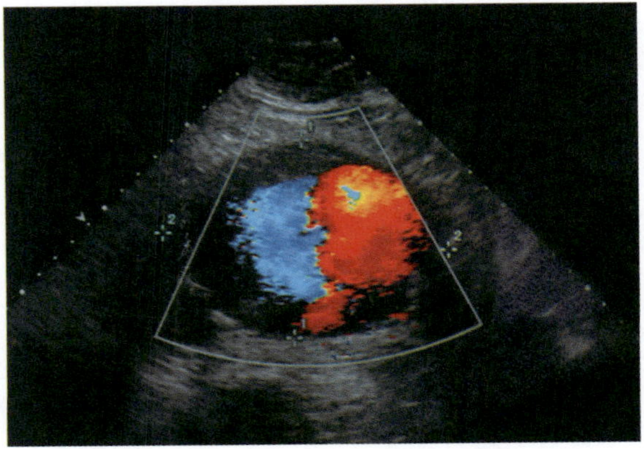

a. a large aneurysm

b. normal multiphasic flow

c. the right/left iliac bifurcation

d. the inferior vena cava to the left of the aorta

A 474

A. A large aneurysm.

The diameter of this aneurysm, were it measured properly in the long axis, would be approximately 9 to 11 cm. Abdominal aortic aneurysms are usually infrarenal, they typically have mural thrombus due to stasis against the wall, and they are most often considered for elective repair when the diameter exceeds 5 to 6 cm.

Q 475

What does this image of the internal carotid artery show?

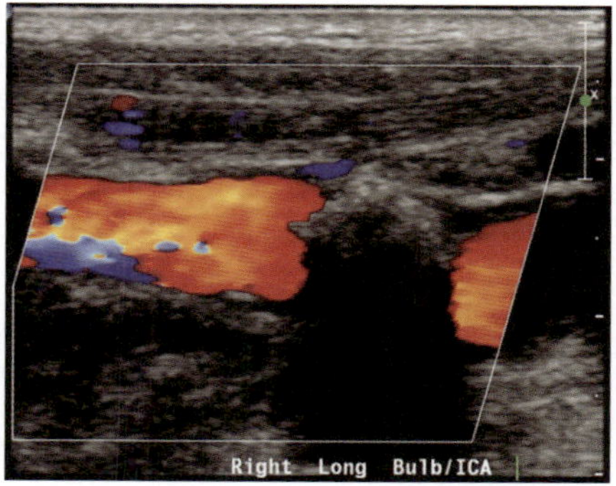

a. carotid body tumor

b. acoustic shadowing

c. extrinsic compression of the ICA

d. ICA occlusion with collateral reconstitution

A 475

B. Acoustic shadowing.

Acoustic shadowing can interfere with both B-mode and color Doppler information, as it does here.

Q 476

You obtain this image from a supraclavicular approach with the beam aimed inferiorly. What does it demonstrate?

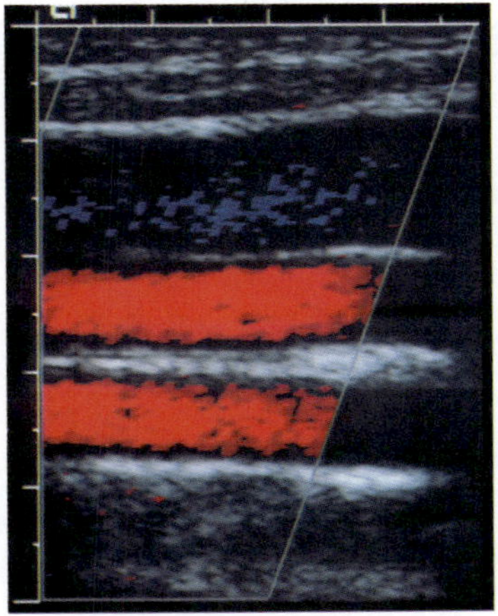

a. retrograde flow in an accessory subclavian vein

b. double subclavian arteries

c. an artifactual image

d. double subclavian veins

A 476

C. An artifactual image.

This artifact–known as doubling–is caused by a strong reflector, in this case the pleura near the clavicle. There is only one subclavian artery, the superior vessel. The deep vessel is its artifactual double.

Q 477

This image of a tortuous internal carotid artery demonstrates all of the following **EXCEPT**:

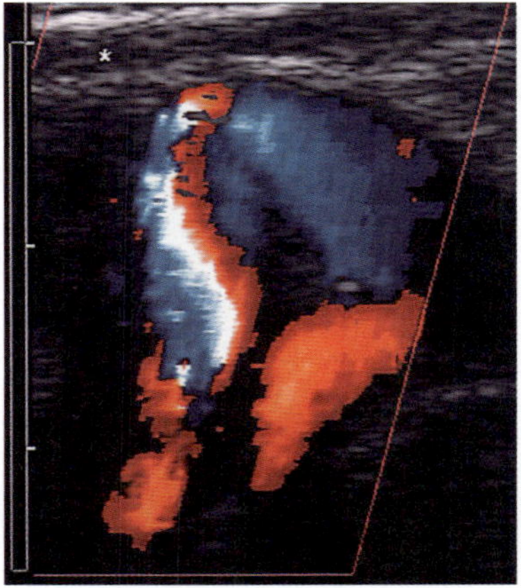

a. a helical flow pattern beyond the tortuosity

b. a stenotic jet

c. faster flow along the outer wall at left

d. aliasing

A 477

B. A stenotic jet is **NOT** demonstrated in this image.

The flow around the tortuosity swirls in a helical pattern. The velocities on the outer wall at left are somewhat higher, creating an aliased blue display with a white area of intermediate velocities in this color flow image. There is no stenosis.

▸ Ridgway DP: *Introduction to Vascular Scanning: A Guide for the Complete Beginner*, 4th edition. Pasadena, Davies Publishing, 2014, pp 388, 392.

Q 478

All of the following statements about this image of the radial/ulnar artery bifurcation are true **EXCEPT**:

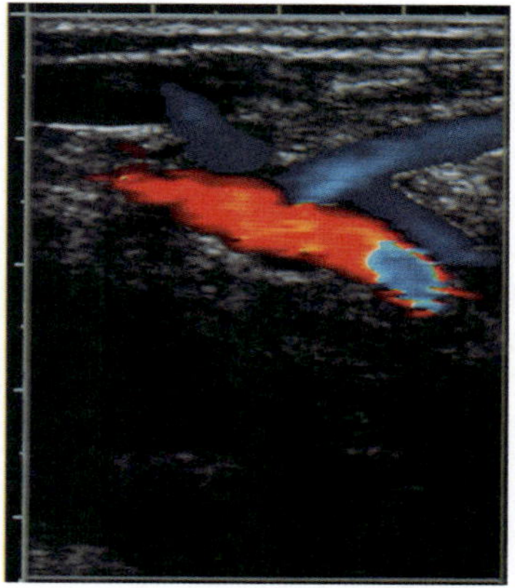

a. The brachial arterial flow is antegrade.

b. The radial arterial flow is antegrade.

c. The ulnar arterial flow is antegrade.

d. The radial arterial flow is retrograde.

A 478

D. This statement–"the radial arterial flow is retrograde"–is **NOT** true.

Everything is normal. The ulnar artery, as usual, dives deeper in the field. Red flow is away from the beam, so the brachial and ulnar arteries are flowing distally (antegrade). Blue is toward the beam, so the radial artery is also flowing distally (antegrade). The brachial vein is partially visualized above the brachial artery and some of the ulnar vein is visible above the ulnar artery. Blue flow is toward the beam because it is moving cephalad.

Q 479

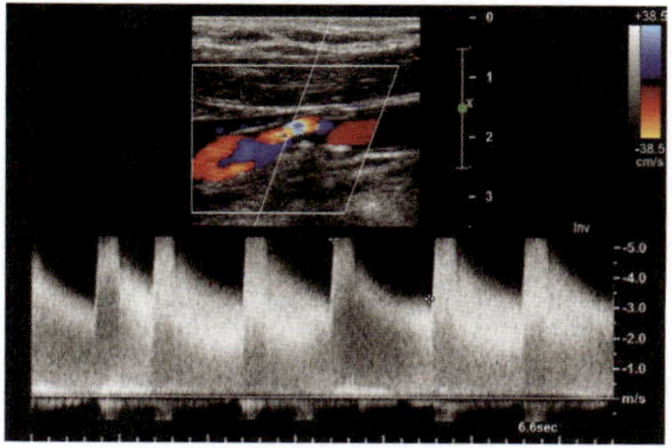

Your patient is having a carotid duplex examination because she wants a second opinion. Her original study is consistent with a high-grade stenosis of her left carotid artery. This image is from your study–it documents a peak systolic velocity (PSV) of 523 cm/sec and an end-diastolic velocity (EDV) of 327 cm/sec. How would you interpret this information?

a. The signal is greater than ½ the pulse repetition frequency, making it nondiagnostic.
b. An accurate PSV can be obtained if the vascular technologist/sonographer uses a high-frequency transducer.
c. The PSV and EDV suggest a 50%–79% diameter reduction based on the University of Washington criteria.
d. The velocity measurements are consistent with a >70% stenosis based on the diagnostic criteria established by the 2003 Society of Radiologists in Ultrasound Consensus Conference.

DAVIES
Registry Reviews & Study Aids

A 479

D. The velocity measurements are consistent with a >70% stenosis based on the diagnostic criteria established by the 2003 Society of Radiologists in Ultrasound Consensus Conference.

▶ Rumwell C, McPharlin M: *Vascular Technology: An Illustrated Review*, 5th edition. Pasadena, Davies Publishing, 2015, pp 234–235.

Q 480

Your patient is a 30-year-old female with a four-day history of calf pain and swelling. This duplex image documents which of the following flow characteristics?

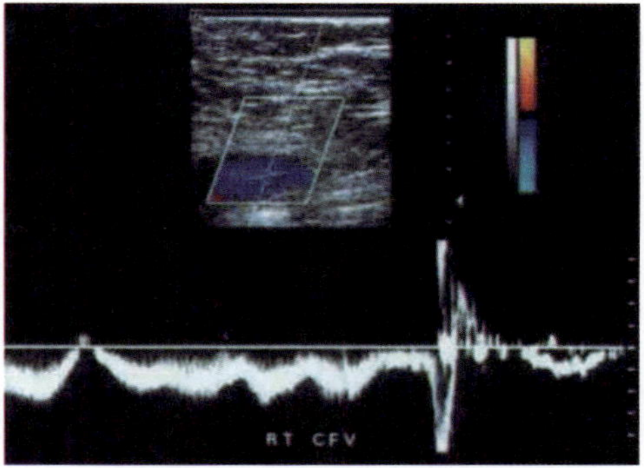

a. pulsatile flow consistent with tricuspid regurgitation

b. venous reflux, suggestive of incompetent valves

c. continuous flow, which implies a proximal obstruction

d. spontaneous, phasic flow, which is within normal limits

A 480

D. Spontaneous, phasic flow, which is within normal limits.

▶ Rumwell C, McPharlin M: *Vascular Technology: An Illustrated Review*, 5th edition. Pasadena, Davies Publishing, 2015, pp 28–29, 36, 303–304.

APPLICATION FOR CME CREDITS

ScoreCards™
for Vascular Technology, 2nd edition

This continuing medical educational (CME) activity is approved for 10 hours of credit by the Society of Diagnostic Medical Sonography. This credit may be applied as follows:

- Sonographers and technologists may apply these hours toward the CME requirements of the ARDMS, ARRT, and/or CCI, as well as to the CME requirements of facilities accredited by the IAC (Vascular Testing).
- Physicians may apply a certain maximum number of SDMS-approved credit hours toward the CME requirements of facilities accredited by the IAC (Vascular Testing). (Be sure to confirm current requirements with the pertinent organizations.) Physicians who are registered sonographers or technologists may apply all of these hours toward the CME requirements of the ARDMS, ARRT, and/or CCI. SDMS-approved credit is not applicable toward the AMA Physician's Recognition Award.
- If you have any questions whatsoever about CME requirements that affect you, please contact the responsible organization directly for current information. CME requirements can and sometimes do change.

DAVIES
Registry Reviews & Study Aids

Objectives of This Activity

Upon completion of this educational activity, you will be able to:

1. Identify the gross anatomy of the central and peripheral arterial and venous systems.
2. Describe the physiology and fluid dynamics of the central and peripheral circulation.
3. Describe how, when, and why imaging and nonimaging techniques are applied to the noninvasive diagnosis of vascular disease.
4. Describe the invasive tests and therapeutic interventions used in vascular disease.
5. List the diagnostic criteria for both imaging and nonimaging tests used in the noninvasive diagnosis of vascular disease.
6. Apply statistical techniques to the analysis of the sensitivity, specificity, accuracy, and negative and positive predictive values of a diagnostic test.

How to Obtain CME Credit

To apply for credit, please do all of the following:

1. Read and study the cards and complete the interactive exercises they contain.
2. Photocopy and complete the following applicant information page, evaluation questionnaire (you grade us!), and CME answer sheet.

3. Return the completed forms together with payment of the administrative and processing fee of $39.50 (if you are the book's original purchaser) or $49.50 (for borrowers) to the following address.

   Davies Publishing, Inc.
   CME Coordinator
   32 South Raymond Avenue, Suite 4
   Pasadena, California 91105-1961

   You can also fax the appropriate pages to 626-792-5308 and pay by credit card. We grade quizzes within 24 hours of receipt and will email your certificate to the email address you provide in your application form. Questions? Please call us at 626-792-3046.

4. If more than one person will be applying for credit, be sure to photocopy the applicant information, evaluation form, and CME quiz so that you always have the original on hand for use.

APPLICANT INFORMATION

ScoreCards for Vascular Technology, 2nd edition

Name ______________________________ Date of Birth ________________

Your degrees and credentials ____

Address ____

City/State/Zip ____

Telephone ________________ Email (required) __________________________

ARDMS# __________ ARRT# __________ SDMS# __________ CCI # __________

Credit Card # _______________________ Exp Date ______ 3- or 4-digit code _____

Name and address on credit card (if different)

____

❑ I purchased this book myself. ❑ I borrowed the book.

Signature and date certifying your completion of the activity

____ Date ________________

NOTE

The original purchaser of this CME activity is entitled to submit this CME application for an administrative fee of $39.50. Please enclose a check payable to Davies Publishing, Inc., or include credit card information with your application. Others may also submit applications for CME credits by completing the activity for an administrative fee of $49.50. The CME administrative fee helps to defray the cost of processing, evaluating, and maintaining a record of your application and the credit you earn. Fees may change without notice. For the current fee, call us at 626-792-3046, email us at cme@daviespublishing.com, or write to us at the aforementioned address. We will be happy to help!

Evaluation—You Grade Us!

Please let us know what you think of the *ScoreCards* study system. Participating in this quality survey is a requirement for CME applicants, and it benefits future readers by ensuring that current readers are satisfied and, if not, that their comments and opinions are heard and taken into account.

1 Why did you purchase *ScoreCards*? (Circle your primary reason.)

Registry review Course text Clinical reference CME activity

2 Have you used *ScoreCards* for other reasons, too? (Circle all that apply.)

Registry review Course text Clinical reference CME activity

3 To what extent did *ScoreCards* meet its stated objectives and your needs? (Circle one.)

Greatly Moderately Minimally Insignificantly

4 The content of *ScoreCards* was (circle one):

Just right Too basic Too advanced

5 The quality of the questions, explanations, illustrations, and case examples was mainly (circle one):

Excellent Good Fair Poor

6 The manner in which *ScoreCards* presents the material is mainly (circle one):

Excellent Good Fair Poor

7 If you used *ScoreCards* to prepare for the registry exam, did you also use other materials or take any exam-preparation courses?

No Yes (please specify what materials and courses)

____

____

8 If you used *ScoreCards* for a course, please list the course name, the instructor's name, the name of the school or program, and any other textbooks you may have used:

Course/Instructor/School or program ________________________

____

9 What did you like best about *ScoreCards*?

____

____

10 What did you like least about *ScoreCards*?

____

____

11 If you used *ScoreCards* to prepare for your registry exam in vascular technology, did you pass?

Yes No Haven't yet taken it

12 May we quote any of your comments in our catalogs or promotional material?

Yes No Further comment

____

____

____

ANSWER SHEET

1. a b c d
2. a b c d
3. a b c d
4. a b c d
5. a b c d
6. a b c d
7. a b c d
8. a b c d
9. a b c d
10. a b c d
11. a b c d
12. a b c d
13. a b c d
14. a b c d
15. a b c d
16. a b c d
17. a b c d
18. a b c d
19. a b c d
20. a b c d
21. a b c d
22. a b c d
23. a b c d
24. a b c d
25. a b c d
26. a b c d
27. a b c d
28. a b c d
29. a b c d
30. a b c d
31. a b c d
32. a b c d
33. a b c d
34. a b c d
35. a b c d
36. a b c d
37. a b c d
38. a b c d
39. a b c d
40. a b c d
41. a b c d
42. a b c d
43. a b c d
44. a b c d
45. a b c d
46. a b c d
47. a b c d
48. a b c d
49. a b c d
50. a b c d
51. a b c d
52. a b c d
53. a b c d
54. a b c d
55. a b c d
56. a b c d
57. a b c d
58. a b c d
59. a b c d
60. a b c d
61. a b c d
62. a b c d
63. a b c d
64. a b c d
65. a b c d
66. a b c d
67. a b c d
68. a b c d
69. a b c d
70. a b c d
71. a b c d
72. a b c d
73. a b c d
74. a b c d
75. a b c d
76. a b c d
77. a b c d
78. a b c d
79. a b c d
80. a b c d
81. a b c d
82. a b c d
83. a b c d
84. a b c d
85. a b c d
86. a b c d
87. a b c d
88. a b c d
89. a b c d
90. a b c d
91. a b c d
92. a b c d
93. a b c d
94. a b c d
95. a b c d
96. a b c d
97. a b c d
98. a b c d
99. a b c d
100. a b c d

CME QUIZ

Please answer the following questions after you have completed the CME activity. There is one best answer for each question. Circle it on the answer sheet on the preceding page. Passing criterion is 70% for attempt 1 and (for those who do not pass on the first attempt) 75% for attempts 2 and 3. Applicants will have no more than 3 attempts to pass.

1. What is the most common anatomic variation of the renal arteries?
   a. retroaortic renal artery
   b. multiple renal arteries
   c. congenital absence of one main renal artery
   d. anterocaval course of right renal artery

2. Which of the following vessels courses along the medial aspect of the psoas muscle?
   a. internal iliac artery
   b. external iliac artery
   c. femoral artery
   d. inferior mesenteric artery

3. The first branch of the external carotid artery is usually the:
   a. facial artery
   b. superficial temporal artery
   c. internal maxillary artery
   d. superior thyroid artery

4. What is the most common anomaly of the circle of Willis?
   a. absence of one of the middle cerebral arteries
   b. duplication of the posterior communicating arteries
   c. hypoplasia of the proximal segment of one of the anterior cerebral arteries
   d. absence or hypoplasia of one or both of the communicating arteries

5. Which vein in the antecubital fossa connects the cephalic and basilic veins?
   a. axillary vein
   b. median cubital vein
   c. cephalic vein
   d. basilic vein

6. Which statement is NOT true regarding the soleal veins?
   a. They empty into the posterior tibial or peroneal veins.
   b. They are found deep in the calf muscle.
   c. They connect with the superficial venous system.
   d. They do not contain valves.

7. Regarding the inferior vena cava, all of the statements below are true EXCEPT:
   a. The inferior vena cava drains into the left atrium of the heart.
   b. The inferior vena cava is formed by the confluence of the common iliac veins.
   c. The inferior vena cava has no valves below the level of its insertion into the heart.
   d. The inferior vena cava courses to the right of the abdominal aorta.

8. The major function of the vasa vasorum is to:
    a. regulate vasodilatation of the arterioles
    b. provide nourishment to the tunica adventitia
    c. provide the major communication in arteriovenous fistulas
    d. provide autoregulation of blood flow to the brain

9. The number of true positives divided by the number of true positives + false positives describes which of the following?
    a. sensitivity
    b. specificity
    c. accuracy
    d. positive predictive value

10. A percentage diameter reduction of 50% in a symmetric narrowing of the carotid artery most closely corresponds to what percentage area reduction?
    a. 35%
    b. 50%
    c. 75%
    d. 90%

11. Arteriovenous fistula is a complication that most commonly occurs with:
    a. reversed vein bypass grafts
    b. in situ grafts
    c. atherectomy
    d. angioplasty

12. A technique in which atherosclerotic plaque is mechanically removed by cutting or pulverizing it and then extracted by suction or downstream embolization is termed:
    a. atherectomy
    b. thrombectomy
    c. angioplasty
    d. endarterectomy

13. What severe symptom of decreased blood perfusion is aggravated by elevation, is relieved by dependency, and often occurs when the patient goes to bed at night?
    a. claudication
    b. cyanosis
    c. rest pain
    d. postprandial pain

14. A nonatherosclerotic, noninflammatory, occlusive, and aneurysmal disorder that primarily affects women and is referred to as a "string of beads" is:
    a. Takayasu's disease
    b. mycotic aneurysm
    c. polyarteritis nodosa
    d. fibromuscular dysplasia

15. The most serious risk from femoropopliteal aneurysms is:
    a. rupture
    b. embolization

c. fistula
d. infection

16. A patient presents to the vascular lab with an abdominal bruit, weight loss, and postprandial pain. Obstruction of which vessel is most likely responsible for these symptoms?
a. renal artery
b. portal vein
c. superior mesenteric artery
d. splenic vein

17. Palpation of a pulse found in the groove behind the medial malleolus of the ankle corresponds to the:
a. posterior tibial artery
b. anterior tibial artery
c. peroneal artery
d. plantar artery

18. An acceleration time of less than 133 msec obtained in the femoral artery suggests:
a. proximal iliac artery stenosis
b. distal femoral artery occlusion
c. pseudoaneurysm of the femoral artery
d. the absence of significant iliac artery disease

19. Reactive hyperemia testing is:
    a. an alternative method to treadmill exercise testing for stressing the peripheral arterial circulation
    b. a method to evaluate the flow patterns within veins
    c. a method utilized in the measurement of limb volume changes
    d. a method to rule out thoracic outlet syndrome

20. What measurement helps in differentiating between inflow and outflow disease by determining the time between the onset of systole and initial (or early) systolic peak?
    a. resistive index
    b. acceleration time
    c. volume flow
    d. A/B ratio

21. Following cessation of exercise in a normal individual, how long does it take for lower extremity blood flow to return to resting values?
    a. 1–5 minutes
    b. 5–10 minutes
    c. 10–15 minutes
    d. as long as 30 minutes

22. Which ABI is indicative of rest pain?
    a. > 1.0
    b. 0.9–1.0
    c. 0.5–0.9
    d. < 0.5

23. Arteriography is contraindicated in a patient with which condition?
    a. diabetes
    b. renal failure
    c. malignancy
    d. vascular disease

24. The biggest contributing risk factor for stroke is:
    a. hypertension
    b. hypercholesterolemia
    c. sedentary life style
    d. alcohol abuse

25. An abnormal sound heard on auscultation caused by flow turbulence is a:
    a. Bernoulli
    b. bruit
    c. Poiseuille
    d. thrill

26. The term *spectral broadening* describes:
    a. the length of the cardiac cycle
    b. a wide range of frequency shifts reflected back to the transducer
    c. a wide-bandwidth continuous-wave Doppler waveform
    d. reversed flow at any point during the cardiac cycle

27. The point at which aliasing occurs in the transmission of a Doppler signal is known as the:
    a. Nyquist limit
    b. Poiseuille's point
    c. Bernoulli's equation
    d. Reynolds number

28. In transcranial Doppler, with the probe placed over the right temporal bone, flow in the right middle cerebral artery will be:
    a. oriented away from the probe
    b. oriented toward the probe
    c. oriented at 90° to the probe
    d. The right middle cerebral artery cannot be visualized from this window.

29. The presence of a mosaic pattern in the color Doppler image of the internal carotid artery most likely indicates:
    a. slow flow proximal to an occlusion
    b. the presence of poststenotic turbulence
    c. reversed flow in the vertebral artery
    d. improper color setup with the pulse repetition frequency set too high

30. Overestimation of the degree of stenosis in the internal carotid artery may be due to all of the following EXCEPT:
    a. increased velocities contralateral to an occlusion
    b. overestimation of the angle of incidence

c. improper location of the sample volume proximal to the stenosis
d. vessel tortuosity

31. Which of the following cannot be determined from an arteriogram?
    a. percent diameter stenosis
    b. reversed flow in the vertebral artery
    c. arterial dissection
    d. flow turbulence

32. Elevated peripheral venous pressure results in:
    a. edema
    b. decreased arterial resistance
    c. lymphangitis
    d. dependent rubor

33. Homan's sign is:
    a. a highly specific sign for lower extremity venous thrombosis
    b. a highly specific sign for upper extremity venous thrombosis
    c. calf discomfort on passive dorsiflexion
    d. numbness of the digits with hyperextension of an extremity

34. In the lower extremity, maximum flow return in the venous system is present with:
    a. inspiration
    b. expiration
    c. Valsalva maneuver
    d. release of distal compression

35. Which of the following describes normal flow in the portal vein?
    a. hepatopetal
    b. hepatofugal
    c. triphasic
    d. bidirectional

36. In duplex sonography, the main purpose of probe compression is to:
    a. rule out incompetent valves
    b. rule out the presence of thrombus
    c. differentiate between superficial and deep veins
    d. differentiate between veins and arteries

37. Which is an advantage of color Doppler imaging over B-mode imaging alone in evaluation of the venous system?
    a. Recanalized thrombi are more readily apparent.
    b. Partially occluding thrombi are better detected.
    c. Venous collaterals are more readily visualized.
    d. All of the above.

38. During the Valsalva maneuver, what happens to pressure in the abdomen and thorax?
    a. intrathoracic pressure increases, abdominal pressure increases
    b. intrathoracic pressure decreases, abdominal pressure decreases
    c. intrathoracic pressure increases, abdominal pressure decreases
    d. intrathoracic pressure decreases, abdominal pressure increases

39. In contrast venography, which finding would indicate the presence of a thrombus?
    a. contrast extravasation
    b. filling defect
    c. increase in opacity
    d. none of the above

40. Symptoms associated with thoracic outlet syndrome include all of the following EXCEPT:
    a. increased blood pressure on the affected side
    b. numbness or tingling of the arm
    c. aching of shoulder and forearm
    d. increased discomfort with upward arm positions

41. A cause of blue toe syndrome is:
    a. venous thrombosis of the pedal veins
    b. hyperemic flow from arteriovenous fistulas
    c. congenital absence of the dorsalis pedis artery
    d. embolization from proximal arteries

42. Which is a complication of dialysis access grafts?
    a. arterial steal
    b. aneurysm
    c. venous stenosis
    d. all of the above

43. The tendency of objects to maintain their status quo is called:
    a. kinetic energy
    b. potential energy
    c. inertia
    d. hydrostatic pressure

44. The term *phasicity*, in reference to the venous system, refers to:
    a. the influence of the cardiac cycle on venous flow
    b. the rate at which the valves open and close
    c. the ebb and flow in the veins that occurs in response to respiration
    d. the effect of intrinsic and extrinsic pressure on venous wall stiffness

45. Which of the following does NOT occur as a result of trauma?
    a. arteriovenous malformation
    b. arteriovenous fistula
    c. pseudoaneurysm
    d. dissection

46. A volume plethysmographic waveform with a normal amplitude, a rounded peak, and an absent dicrotic notch is most likely indicative of:
    a. arterial disease proximal to the level of tracing
    b. arterial occlusion at the level of tracing
    c. normal arterial inflow
    d. arterial disease distal to the level of tracing

47. How much of the body's blood volume is found in the veins at any moment?
    a. 40%–50%
    b. 60%–75%
    c. 10%–20%
    d. 25%–64%

48. The degree of stenosis in the internal carotid artery can be determined by all of the following parameters EXCEPT:
    a. ICA/CCA ratio
    b. heart rate
    c. peak frequency shift
    d. peak systolic velocity

49. The vein that normally courses between the superior mesenteric artery and the abdominal aorta is the:
    a. inferior mesenteric vein
    b. superior mesenteric vein
    c. portal vein
    d. left renal vein

50. Ankle systolic pressure, in a normal study, should be:
    a. equal to the lowest brachial blood pressure
    b. less than the highest brachial blood pressure
    c. less than the right brachial blood pressure
    d. the same as or greater than the highest brachial blood pressure

51. Why do collateral vessels tend to have higher resistance than normal flow channels?
    a. higher viscosity
    b. small lumen diameter
    c. greater length
    d. small lumen diameter and greater length

52. An aneurysm resulting from infection is called:
    a. mycotic
    b. ectatic
    c. saccular
    d. fusiform

53. A late complication of extremity bypass grafts is:
    a. hematoma
    b. pseudoaneurysm
    c. intimal hyperplasia
    d. arteriovenous fistula

54. What should an examiner do if the great saphenous vein is NOT identified at the appropriate location?
    a. use a lateral approach
    b. use a posterior approach
    c. increase probe pressure
    d. decrease probe pressure

55. The diagnostic test that most readily differentiates between primary ischemic and primary hemorrhagic stroke is:
    a. duplex ultrasonography
    b. electrocardiogram
    c. computed tomography of the brain
    d. magnetic resonance angiography

56. In the posterolateral aspect of the carotid bulb, helical flow with flow separation is a sign of:
    a. stenosis
    b. normal flow dynamics
    c. thrombosis
    d. dissection

57. Which artery is likely to be enlarged in the presence of vertebral artery occlusion?
    a. contralateral vertebral
    b. ipsilateral external carotid
    c. ipsilateral subclavian
    d. contralateral internal thoracic

58. A disease that occurs predominantly in male smokers that involves thrombosis of the small or medium-sized arteries of the extremities is:
    a. Allen's disease
    b. Raynaud's disease
    c. Buerger's disease
    d. thoracic outlet disease

59. A loss of the triphasic waveform in the popliteal artery can be caused by:
    a. exercise
    b. proximal occlusion
    c. distal vasodilatation
    d. all of the above

60. What happens to pressure in the abdomen and thorax during inspiration?
    a. Intrathoracic pressure increases, abdominal pressure decreases.
    b. Intrathoracic pressure decreases, abdominal pressure increases.
    c. Intrathoracic pressure decreases, abdominal pressure decreases.
    d. Intrathoracic pressure increases, abdominal pressure increases.

61. What would occur to the pressure gradient across an arterial segment in which the radius has been reduced by 1/2, according to Poiseuille's law?
    a. decrease
    b. no effect
    c. increase
    d. not enough information to determine

62. All of the following statements regarding intrathoracic pressure are true EXCEPT:
    a. Intrathoracic pressure is increased with the Valsalva maneuver.
    b. Intrathoracic pressure is increased with inspiration.
    c. Intrathoracic pressure has a major effect on venous return.
    d. Venous return from the upper extremities is reduced when intrathoracic pressure is high.

63. Which of the following techniques would be most helpful in performing a vein mapping of the saphenous vein?
   a. Use a high-frequency probe and light probe pressure to track the saphenous vein.
   b. Place the patient in a prone position to improve access to the saphenous vein.
   c. Decrease the room temperature so the small saphenous vein will become dilated.
   d. Place the patient in an upright position to improve visualization of the saphenous vein.

64. How should a patient be positioned to obtain digital pressures of the toes?
   a. decubitus
   b. standing
   c. Trendelenburg
   d. supine

65. All of the following are consistent with the diagnosis of right internal carotid artery occlusion EXCEPT:
   a. debris-filled right internal carotid artery
   b. increased diastolic flow in the ipsilateral common carotid artery
   c. low-resistance flow in the right external carotid artery
   d. hyperemic flow in the left common carotid artery

66. The arterial supply to carotid body tumors is primarily from the:
   a. vasa vasorum of the internal carotid artery
   b. vertebral artery
   c. thyrocervical trunk
   d. branches of the external carotid artery

67. The basilar artery divides into the:
    a. posterior cerebral arteries
    b. vertebral arteries
    c. posterior communicating arteries
    d. posterior inferior cerebellar arteries

68. Atherosclerosis in the cerebrovascular system most commonly occurs in the:
    a. innominate artery
    b. left subclavian artery
    c. intracranial internal carotid artery
    d. carotid bulb

69. All of the following are paired veins EXCEPT:
    a. peroneal
    b. radial
    c. cephalic
    d. posterior tibial

70. Which vessel is evaluated from the foramen magnum window with transcranial Doppler?
    a. posterior cerebral artery
    b. posterior communicating artery
    c. basilar artery
    d. anterior communicating artery

71. Lymphedema is a result of:
    a. incompetent venous valves
    b. impaired transport of lymph
    c. deep venous thrombosis
    d. chronic venous insufficiency

72. In CW Doppler studies, a continuous venous signal is commonly seen with:
    a. collateral flow
    b. fluid overload
    c. congestive heart failure
    d. normality

73. The ankle/brachial index is calculated by dividing the ankle pressure by the:
    a. highest of the two brachial pressures
    b. lowest of the two brachial pressures
    c. right brachial pressure
    d. left brachial pressure

74. A typical venous Doppler waveform obtained proximal to an arteriovenous fistula can be described as being/having:
    a. unchanged from normal
    b. prominent respiratory phasicity
    c. continuous low velocity
    d. increased velocity and pulsatility

75. If the noninvasive test results are positive but the gold standard shows normal results, the noninvasive test results are referred to as:
    a. true positive
    b. false positive
    c. true negative
    d. false negative

76. Which component of the reflected signals does power Doppler encode?
    a. frequency shift
    b. velocity
    c. amplitude
    d. wavelength

77. In pulsed-wave Doppler studies, loss of the spectral window characterizes which type of blood flow?
    a. flow turbulence
    b. parabolic flow
    c. laminar flow
    d. all of the above

78. The greatest clinical danger from venous thrombosis is:
    a. pulmonary embolism
    b. superficial venous obstruction
    c. venous hypertension
    d. incompetent valves

79. What factor has the greatest influence on flow resistance?
    a. viscosity
    b. vessel radius
    c. vessel length
    d. pressure gradient

80. Virchow's triad consists of three factors that are significant in the development of venous thrombosis. These are:
    a. stasis, hypercoagulability, extrinsic compression
    b. hypercoagulability, cancer, stasis
    c. stasis, extrinsic compression, trauma
    d. trauma, stasis, hypercoagulability

81. The Bernoulli effect describes:
    a. decreased resistance distal to a stenosis
    b. decreased pressure in regions of high flow speed
    c. decreased velocities in regions of flow turbulence
    d. decreased flow volume in critical stenosis

82. Which vessel normally exhibits a triphasic waveform?
    a. common carotid artery
    b. vertebral artery
    c. subclavian artery
    d. internal carotid artery

83. What is the most common cause of portal hypertension in the United States?
    a. schistosomiasis
    b. cirrhosis
    c. hyperlipidemia
    d. hypertension

84. The most common cause of upper extremity venous thrombus is:
    a. weightlifting
    b. blunt trauma
    c. pregnancy
    d. intravenous catheters and lines

85. Inferior vena cava thrombosis most likely results in:
    a. swelling of the right lower extremity only
    b. bilateral swelling of the lower extremities
    c. unilateral calf vein swelling
    d. abdominal cavity swelling

86. A 53-year-old male presents to the vascular lab with a six-month history of severe hypertension and abdominal bruit. Which vessel is most likely the source of the patient's symptoms?
    a. superior mesenteric artery
    b. celiac trunk
    c. renal artery
    d. hepatic artery

87. Which of the following is NOT a symptom of pulmonary embolism?
    a. dyspnea
    b. chest pain
    c. tachycardia
    d. claudication

88. Which of the following is a sign of chronic venous insufficiency?
    a. dyspnea
    b. shooting pains in the extremity
    c. numbness
    d. hyperpigmentation

89. Which of the following is NOT a contraindication for treadmill stress testing?
    a. history of cardiac problems
    b. history of stroke
    c. history of claudication
    d. shortness of breath

90. With calf compression, augmentation of the Doppler signal in the femoral vein indicates:
    a. reflux
    b. incompetent valves
    c. deep venous thrombosis in the popliteal vein
    d. normality

91. Which finding is NOT associated with venous ulcers?
    a. brawny discoloration
    b. shiny skin
    c. location near medial malleolus
    d. irregular borders

92. The Reynolds number denotes the:
    a. effect of pressure on volume flow
    b. effect of arteriolar vasodilation or vasoconstriction on flow velocity
    c. point at which resistance to flow is increased in a stenosis
    d. point at which flow becomes turbulent

93. What is the most common anatomic location of renal allografts?
    a. left iliac fossa
    b. right iliac fossa
    c. mid pelvis
    d. Morison's pouch

94. The saphenofemoral junction is identified by duplex sonography:
    a. at the level of the knee
    b. at the mid thigh
    c. in the adductor canal
    d. near the inguinal ligament

95. Which of the following refers to neurologic symptoms that are of short duration, completely resolving in less than 24 hours?
    a. CVA
    b. RIND
    c. TIA
    d. HTN

96. What is the main power source for blood propulsion in the venous system?
    a. bicuspid valves
    b. right atrium
    c. calf muscle
    d. respiration

97. A unilateral temporary vision loss associated with cerebrovascular disease is known as:
    a. dysphasia
    b. amaurosis fugax
    c. diplopia
    d. ataxia

98. How should the patient be positioned to facilitate visualization of varicose veins?
    a. standing
    b. supine
    c. Trendelenburg
    d. prone

99. Which physical finding is seen with arterial insufficiency more frequently than with venous stasis?
    a. red or blue skin
    b. pallor
    c. brown skin discoloration
    d. induration

100. Under which of the following conditions will you see increased diastolic flow in the superior mesenteric artery?
    a. postprandial state
    b. stenosis
    c. replaced hepatic artery
    d. all of the above

SCORECARDS QUESTIONS CROSS-REFERENCED TO THE ARDMS EXAM CONTENT OUTLINE

Note: *For your convenience, ScoreCards questions are arranged according to the topics and subtopics covered on the ARDMS exam (see www.ardms.org).*

NORMAL ANATOMY, PERFUSION, AND FUNCTION—21%

Evaluate normal anatomy, perfusion, and function

Aortoiliac vasculature: *See questions* 1, 2, 3, 4, 11, 12, 40, 41, 42, 48, 49, 56, 70, 93, 438, 439, 440, 442.

Upper extremity veins: *See questions* 28, 29, 30, 31, 43, 44, 45, 53, 54, 175, 188, 460.

Lower extremity veins: *See questions* 32, 33, 36, 37, 39, 43, 44, 45, 163, 167, 168, 169, 170, 171, 184, 186, 187, 188, 402, 403, 404, 405, 438, 461, 467, 468, 480.

Native upper extremity arteries: *See questions* 3, 24, 41, 42, 46, 106, 348, 460, 478.

Native lower extremity arteries: *See questions* 4, 7, 8, 41, 42, 46, 170, 222, 276, 438, 461.

Mesenteric vasculature: *See questions* 9, 39, 291, 293, 308, 442, 451, 464.

Renal vasculature: *See questions* 5, 6, 10, 35, 55, 305, 322, 442, 445, 446, 451, 453, 457.

Hepatoportal system: *See questions* 34, 38, 39, 50, 51, 52, 440, 441, 455, 457.

Inferior vena cava and/or iliac veins: *See questions* 39, 40, 44, 445, 451, 457.

Extracranial cerebrovascular system: *See questions* 1, 2, 13, 14, 15, 16, 17, 18, 19, 20, 21, 22, 23, 25, 26, 27, 47, 100, 108, 109, 470.

Intracranial cerebrovascular exams (transcranial Doppler (TCD) and transcranial imaging (TCI): *See questions* 93, 94, 95, 96, 110, 111, 113, 114, 115.

Vein mapping: *See questions* 329, 330, 331, 355.

PATHOLOGY, PERFUSION, AND FUNCTION—32%

Evaluate pathology, perfusion, and function

Aortoiliac disease (atherosclerosis, aneurysm, dissection, etc.): *See questions* 67, 79, 130, 131, 207, 211, 212, 230, 273, 352, 353, 421, 423, 427.

Venous insufficiency: *See questions* 141, 142, 147, 149, 151, 153, 154, 155, 156, 157, 158, 162, 164, 165, 167, 176, 179, 187, 191, 192, 197, 200, 201, 202, 217, 301, 330, 414.

Upper extremity venous disease (thrombosis, thoracic outlet syndrome, extrinsic compression, etc.): *See questions* 143, 147, 175, 350, 351.

Lower extremity venous disease (thrombosis, extrinsic compression, etc.): *See questions* 136, 137, 138, 139, 140, 141, 142, 144, 145, 146, 147, 148, 149, 152, 153, 154, 155, 158, 159, 173, 179, 180, 187, 189, 190, 193, 194, 201, 202, 414, 424.

Native upper extremity artery disease (atherosclerosis, aneurysm, dissection, thoracic outlet syndrome, etc.): *See questions* 24, 62, 64, 75, 83, 207, 211, 212, 214, 218, 220, 275.

Native lower extremity artery disease (atherosclerosis, aneurysm, dissection, extrinsic compression, etc.): *See questions* 203, 207, 208, 210, 211, 212, 213, 217, 218, 224, 225, 226, 227, 231, 247, 271, 272, 277, 278, 281, 282, 284, 286, 287, 447, 448, 458, 471.

Mesenteric vasculature disease (atherosclerosis, aneurysm, dissection, thrombosis, extrinsic compression, etc.): *See questions* 208, 211, 212, 293, 299, 307, 310.

Renal vasculature disease (atherosclerosis, aneurysm, dissection, thrombosis, extrinsic compression, fibromuscular dysplasia, etc.): *See questions* 127, 208, 211, 212, 289, 292, 296, 297, 303, 304, 306, 311, 312, 321, 323, 472, 474.

Hepatoportal system disease (thrombosis, Budd-Chiari syndrome, portal hypertension, etc.): *See questions* 290, 295, 298, 300, 301, 313, 314, 315, 319, 320, 323, 420, 431, 432, 436, 437, 444.

Inferior vena cava and/or iliac vein disease (thrombosis, extrinsic compression, etc.): *See questions* 39, 40, 50, 152, 153, 182, 321, 436, 445, 451, 452, 457.

Extracranial cerebrovascular disease: *See questions* 21, 82, 83, 84, 86, 97, 116, 349, 462, 463.

Intracranial cerebrovascular disease (TCD and TCI) (stroke, vasospasm, agitated saline for patent foramen ovale (PFO), intraoperative emboli monitoring, etc.): *See questions* 57, 58, 60, 61, 62, 63, 64, 65, 66, 67, 68, 69, 70, 72, 73, 74, 75, 76, 77, 78, 81, 89, 92, 111, 115, 116, 117, 123, 124, 125, 129, 134, 211, 422, 454, 473, 477, 479.

Incidental findings (thyroid mass, Baker cyst, carotid body tumor, etc.): *See questions* 59, 60, 61, 132, 185, 203, 204, 205, 206, 209, 215, 216, 219, 220, 223, 408, 453, 456, 459.

Critical findings (aneurysm, acute deep vein thrombosis, critical stenosis, etc.): *See questions* 66, 68, 139, 147, 148, 149, 159, 203, 205, 207, 210, 213, 295, 325, 334, 335, 340, 349, 352, 353, 354, 416, 419.

SURGICALLY ALTERED ANATOMY AND PATHOLOGY—6%

Evaluate surgically altered anatomy and pathology

Dialysis access: *See questions* 341, 342, 343, 356, 357, 358, 359, 360, 361, 418.

Post intervention (endovascular, aneurysm repair (EVAR), inferior vane cava (IVC) filter, venous ablation, bypass grafts, transjugular intrahepatic portosystemic shunt (TIPS), stents, etc.): *See questions* 71, 88, 135, 209, 220, 224, 225, 228, 229, 230, 231, 232, 233, 256, 257, 258, 259, 260, 262, 266, 286, 294, 316, 324, 325, 326, 333, 335, 340, 341, 342, 343, 344, 347, 356, 357, 358, 359, 360, 361, 418, 452, 465, 469.

Transplanted organs: *See questions* 294, 309, 344.

PHYSIOLOGIC EXAMINATIONS—12%

Perform physiologic arterial examinations

Arteriovenous physiology: *See questions* 415, 416, 417, 419.

Manually calculate pressure indices (ankle-brachial index (ABI), segmental pressures, etc.): *See questions* 226, 239, 243, 244, 245, 246, 247, 248, 252, 263, 265, 271, 272, 273, 274, 279, 280, 281, 285, 346.

Obtain appropriate diagnostic waveforms/pressures with and without provocative/exercise maneuvers: *See questions* 75, 84, 85, 87, 90, 9, 112, 116, 121, 122, 124, 125, 126, 127, 128, 210, 221, 222, 226, 232, 237, 245, 246, 249, 251, 263, 270, 277, 283, 285, 336, 337, 391, 425.

Select appropriate instrumentation (photoplethysmography (PPG), sensors, cuffs, presets, protocols, etc.): *See questions* 237, 240, 241, 245, 251, 253, 263, 275.

Perform physiologic venous examinations

Venous physiology: *See questions* 400, 401, 402, 403, 404, 405, 406, 407, 409, 410, 411, 412, 413, 414.

Obtain appropriate venous photoplethysmography (PPG) diagnostic waveforms (with and without tourniquets; plantar flexion and dorsiflexion): *See questions* 150, 189, 200, 201, 202, 314, 315, 409.

Select appropriate venous photoplethysmography (PPG) instrumentation (sensors, presets, protocols, etc.): *See questions* 189, 200, 201, 202, 240, 245, 253.